Healthy Eating Policy and Political Philosophy

Healthy Eating Policy and Political Philosophy

A Public Reason Approach

ANNE BARNHILL AND MATTEO BONOTTI

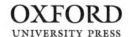

OXFORD
UNIVERSITY PRESS

OXFORD
UNIVERSITY PRESS

Oxford University Press is a department of the University of Oxford. It furthers
the University's objective of excellence in research, scholarship, and education
by publishing worldwide. Oxford is a registered trade mark of Oxford University
Press in the UK and certain other countries.

Published in the United States of America by Oxford University Press
198 Madison Avenue, New York, NY 10016, United States of America.

© Oxford University Press 2022

Library of Congress Control Number: 2021029413
ISBN 978-0-19-093788-1

DOI: 10.1093/oso/9780190937881.001.0001

1 3 5 7 9 8 6 4 2

Printed by Integrated Books International, United States of America

Contents

Acknowledgements

An earlier draft of this book was presented at a workshop held at the University of Milan in February 2020. We are very grateful to Emilio D'Orazio (Director of POLITEIA—Centro per la ricerca e la formazione in politica ed etica) and to Culinary Mind—Centre for the Philosophy of Food for organizing the event, and to Giulia Bistagnino, Andrea Borghini, John Coggon, Matilde Pileri, Nicola Piras, Beatrice Serini, Federico Zuolo, and all other workshop attendees for their extensive and constructive feedback. We would also like to thank Justin Bernstein, Paul Billingham, Rebecca Brown, Diana Burnett, Carol Devine, Jonathan Herington, Lotte Holm, Michele Loi, Jocelyn Maclure, Mary C. Rawlinson, Ben Saunders, Andreas Schmidt, Ian Werkheiser and audiences at Cardiff University, the Centre de recherche en éthique de l'Université de Montréal (CRÉUM), Johns Hopkins University, the Eighth International Conference on Food Studies (2018), University of British Columbia, and the University of Texas–Rio Grande Valley for their comments on early draft chapters. The idea for this book originated from the workshop Promoting Health through Food Policy in Diverse Societies, held at Cardiff University on 14–15 September 2016 and funded by a homonymous Wellcome Trust Society & Ethics Small Grant (Wellcome Trust reference 203779/Z/16/Z). We would like to thank the Wellcome Trust for their support. Furthermore, Matteo Bonotti's work on this book was supported in part by the grant Civic Virtue in Public Life: Understanding and Countering Incivility in Liberal Democracies, funded as part of the Self, Virtue and Public Life Project, a three-year research initiative based at the Institute for the Study of Human Flourishing at the University of Oklahoma, funded with generous support from the Templeton Religion Trust. Matteo Bonotti is also very grateful to his family for their constant love and support. He dedicates this book to his grandmothers, Rosalba and Urania, whose cooking accompanied some of the best moments of his childhood. Anne Barnhill dedicates this book to her daughters, Athena and Adeline, who bring both conscience and gusto to what they eat.

Parts of this book draw on published journal articles. Chapter 3 draws on Matteo Bonotti (2013), 'Legislating about Unhealthy Food: A Millian

Approach', *Ethical Perspectives*, 20 (4): 555–89, doi: 10.2143/EP.20.4.3005350. We are grateful to Peeters Publishers for permission to reprint material from this article. Chapter 5 draws on Matteo Bonotti and Anne Barnhill (2019), 'Are Healthy Eating Policies Consistent with Public Reason?', *Journal of Applied Philosophy*, 36 (3): 506–22, doi: 10.1111/japp.12318. We are grateful to John Wiley & Sons Ltd for permission to reprint material from this article. Finally, we would like to thank Peter Ohlin, Paloma Escovedo, Archanaa Raja and Saloni Vohra for their constant support and advice throughout the book manuscript preparation and production process.

Introduction

Rethinking Healthy Eating Policy

Contemporary states are becoming increasingly interventionist in matters of public health, including when it comes to efforts aimed at changing people's dietary habits, such as soda taxes and food bans. These kinds of measures have been criticized, both by members of the public and by scholars. Many of these criticisms have been driven by the view that efforts aimed at improving people's dietary choices are instances of government paternalism, that is efforts aiming to make people better off that are motivated by a negative judgment about the individual and/or interfere with their freedom without their consent (Dworkin 2020; Quong 2011). Among public health ethicists and philosophers, much debate has been conducted along these lines, with some defending the permissibility of paternalistic healthy eating efforts and others criticizing them on various grounds.

This debate is interesting but we think that its dominance pays short shrift to other key issues in the ethical assessment of healthy eating efforts, namely issues related to respecting diverse conceptions of the good and diverse perspectives and practices vis-à-vis eating and health. In this book, we argue that in order to respect this diversity, healthy eating efforts should be publicly justified based on public reasons, reasons that all citizens[1] of a liberal society could accept at some level of idealization despite their diverse conceptions of the good. We defend a specific version of public reason, i.e. 'accessibility', and explain how it can help us to critically assess existing and proposed healthy eating efforts. We conclude by providing a framework that public health practitioners and other stakeholders could use to analyse healthy eating efforts, to ensure that the latter are publicly justified—i.e. justified based on reasons that all citizens could accept despite their diverse conceptions of the good.

---

[1] Throughout the book, we use the term 'citizen' broadly to also include those who reside in a country and are affected by its laws but are not legal citizens of that country.

Healthy Eating Policy and Political Philosophy. Anne Barnhill and Matteo Bonotti, Oxford University Press. © Oxford University Press 2022. DOI: 10.1093/oso/9780190937881.003.0001

The central thread of this book is therefore to develop a 'public reason approach' to healthy eating policy: to consider how a dominant and fruitful approach in political philosophy (public reason) applies to healthy eating efforts, and to develop a concrete tool (the framework presented in Chapter 7) that can be used in the assessment of actual healthy eating efforts. We take, as it were, a 'farm to fork' approach to the ethics of healthy eating efforts: we engage with rather abstract theories and debates in political philosophy, consider the implications of different theoretical positions for healthy eating efforts, and then develop a concrete tool that can be used in real-world policymaking.

Along with developing this 'public reason approach' to healthy eating efforts, this book is also meant to serve another purpose: to bring not just public reason but political philosophy more generally to bear on healthy eating efforts and the debates about them. We hope this will be of interest to two audiences. The first consists of those who are familiar with healthy eating efforts but may have little experience with political philosophy—e.g. public health researchers and practitioners, some public health ethicists, and other researchers who take an interest in healthy eating efforts. This book will provide them with an introduction to how concepts, theories, and debates from political philosophy bear on healthy eating efforts and the ongoing controversies about them. We recommend that this audience focus their energy on Chapters 1, 2, 4, and 7. The second audience comprises political philosophers, who will be already familiar with the concepts and theoretical debates we consider but may find their concrete application to healthy eating efforts to be of interest.

Our analysis in the book proceeds as follows. Chapter 1 lays the ground-work for the rest of the book. It introduces healthy eating efforts and briefly illustrates some ethical objections to them. The chapter also outlines a conception of eating and food experiences that underlies the book: food and eating have many kinds of value for individuals, families, and communities, and the value of food and eating can be both positive and negative. Healthy eating can result in trade-offs between different valued ends, such that people face dilemmas related to food, eating, and health. Central to this chapter and to the overall book is the claim that when particular healthy eating efforts are envisioned, public health policymakers should consider how such efforts may affect citizens in the context of their lives, given the importance that food, eating, and health (as well as other values) can have for them.

Chapter 2 illustrates the implications of key debates on justice in political philosophy for the analysis of healthy eating efforts. This chapter may be especially interesting to readers who are not familiar with key concepts and theories in political philosophy. The chapter first considers different conceptions of freedom in political philosophy, including negative, positive, and republican freedom (or freedom as non-domination). It then examines the idea of democracy, and especially the difference between aggregative (i.e. vote-centric) and deliberative conceptions. Furthermore, the chapter considers different conceptions of equality and justice as well as theories of multiculturalism. Finally, it introduces the debate on state neutrality and perfectionism, which is central to the rest of the book. For each of these issues in political philosophy, the chapter examines their relationship with healthy eating efforts.

Chapter 3 zooms in on John Stuart Mill's liberalism, examining its implications for healthy eating efforts. This analysis is relevant to the book's argument for a number of reasons. First, Mill is one of the key representatives of perfectionist liberalism, a strand in liberalism that is centred around the value of individual autonomy and the importance for the state to legislate in ways that advance citizens' autonomous flourishing in all aspects of their lives. Second, efforts targeting unhealthy dietary patterns are often criticized for being paternalistic, and Mill is perhaps the archetype of a liberal anti-paternalist thinker (e.g. see Saunders 2013). Indeed his ideas are often appealed to by critics of state paternalism (Powers et al. 2012), including those who challenge healthy eating efforts.

Chapter 4 introduces and critically examines debates about paternalism and healthy eating efforts in bioethics and political philosophy. These debates normally emphasize views about autonomy, including controversial substantive views about the importance of autonomy. We focus instead on an objection to paternalism advanced by Jonathan Quong (2011), which is not rooted in a controversial view about the importance of autonomy but instead in John Rawls's (2005a) demand that citizens ought to be regarded as free and equal and as capable of forming, revising, and rationally pursuing a conception of the good. We critically assess Quong's view in relation to healthy eating efforts. Contrary to Quong, who argues that the Rawlsian normative ideal requires policymakers to assume that citizens always behave rationally, we contend that regarding citizens as free and equal requires instead recognizing and respecting their diverse conceptions of the good and diverse perspectives and practices vis-à-vis eating and health.

Chapter 5 applies a public reason approach to healthy eating efforts. Public reason is the view that state laws and policies can rightly be implemented only if they are justified on the basis of reasons that are 'public reasons,' i.e. reasons that all citizens can accept at some level of idealization despite their different conceptions of the good. This chapter asks when, if ever, healthy eating efforts are publicly justified and consistent with the idea of public reason. First, the chapter provides an account of various ways in which reasonable pluralism is relevant to the analysis of public reason in relation to healthy eating efforts. By drawing on some of the analysis conducted in previous chapters, it especially illustrates the existence of different conceptions of health, different levels of priority assigned to health as opposed to other values, and different kinds of social and cultural importance assigned to eating practices. The chapter then introduces three major conceptions of public reason—'shareability', 'intelligibility', and 'accessibility'—and applies them to healthy eating efforts. The chapter concludes that healthy eating efforts are consistent with public reason only under the 'accessibility' conception.

Chapter 6 employs the accessibility conception of public reason to critically assess healthy eating efforts in liberal democracies and identify respects in which these efforts and objections to them may be unreasonable, i.e. publicly unjustified and therefore illegitimate. In order to do so, it disaggregates the concept of 'evaluative standards' that is central to the accessibility conception of public reason in order to develop a categorization of evaluative standards that allows us to explain in what sense different types of healthy eating efforts may be unreasonable.

Chapter 7 develops an ethics framework that can be used by public health policymakers and others to help them navigate the complex empirical and moral issues surrounding healthy eating efforts discussed in the previous chapters. It poses questions that those designing, modifying, or assessing healthy eating efforts should ask about such efforts, in order to ensure that the efforts comply with the demands of public reason. The chapter also highlights the need for a multilayered approach to healthy eating policy involving community-based forums, consultation procedures, and deliberative settings.

Lastly, we conclude the book by summarizing the book's key themes and outlining important areas for future research at the intersection of political philosophy and food policy.

1

The Ethical Dilemmas of
(Un)Healthy Eating

1.1. Introduction

This chapter lays the groundwork for the rest of the book. It provides an in-
troductory overview of healthy eating efforts and briefly surveys some ethical objections to them. The chapter also lays out a conception of eating and
food experiences that underlies this book's analysis: food and eating have
many kinds of value for individuals, families, and communities, both positive and negative. Healthy eating can involve trade-offs between different
valued ends, and people can find themselves in dilemmas surrounding food,
eating, and health. For example, a mother at the end of a busy day might face
this dilemma: do I cook a healthier dinner for my kids (which they might not
like and might not eat, and which might lead to friction at dinner time), or
do I spend that time helping my kids with their homework and talking with
them about their day, and feed them a not-very-healthy frozen pizza heated
up in the microwave? Less healthy dietary patterns can represent a person's
best effort to respond to the dilemmas and trade-offs that she experiences in
the context of her life.

This does not mean that we must assume that unhealthy dietary patterns[1]
always represent the best response to trade-offs and dilemmas around eating.
It is reasonable for public health policymakers to assume that many people's
unhealthy dietary patterns are misaligned with their life plans, and to assume that making their dietary patterns healthier would make many people
better off. But this assumption gets public health only so far. When particular
healthy eating efforts are envisioned, it is important to consider how those

---

[1] By 'unhealthy dietary patterns' we mean dietary patterns associated with significantly higher
risk of diet-related illness, as compared to dietary patterns that conform with health-based dietary
recommendations.

Healthy Eating Policy and Political Philosophy. Anne Barnhill and Matteo Bonotti, Oxford University Press. © Oxford
University Press 2022. DOI: 10.1093/oso/9780190937881.003.0002

particular efforts may affect the target population in the context of their lives, given what food, eating and health mean to them.

1.2. The public health problem of dietary patterns

'Unhealthy diet is the leading risk factor for deaths in the majority of countries in the world.'[2] These are the words of Ashkan Afshin (quoted in Aubrey 2019), the lead author of a major 2019 study examining the impact of unhealthy diet on people's mortality and morbidity (Afshin et al. 2019). The study concluded that in 2017, 11 million deaths and 255 million DALYs (disability-adjusted life years, a measure of disease and disability) were attributable to diet, and that improving diets could reduce the number of deaths by 20% globally. The authors found that the major risk factors related to diet were high consumption of sodium, low consumption of whole grains, and low consumption of fruits. In the United States, e.g., 91% of people do not consume the recommended amounts of fruit and vegetable, and most people consume more than the recommended amounts of sodium and added sugar (Lee-Kwan et al. 2017, p. 66).

The problem of unhealthy dietary patterns is closely related to the problem of overweight and obesity, which are caused by both diet and physical activity; more precisely, by the excessive consumption of calories relative to energy expenditure. Overweight and obesity rates have increased dramatically worldwide since the 1980s. In 2016, 39% of adults worldwide were overweight; 13% were obese (World Health Organization [WHO] 2017). In some countries, rates were significantly higher; e.g. in the US 39.6% of adults and 18.5% of youth were obese in 2015–16, with higher rates amongst some racial/ethnic minorities (Hales et al. 2018). According to public health organizations and experts, these high overweight and obesity rates have considerable consequences for public health, increasing risk for diet-related disease; Lim et al. (2013) conclude that overweight and obesity resulted in an estimated 3.4 million deaths worldwide in 2010.

To many researchers and policymakers, this 'epidemic' of unhealthy diet, overweight, and obesity demands a comprehensive response by public health policymakers and the global community more generally (Institute of Medicine [IOM] and Committee on Accelerating Progress in Obesity

---

[2] This section draws on Barnhill (2019) and Barnhill et al. (2018).

Prevention [CAPOP] 2012; Swinburn et al. 2019; WHO 2013). However, many of the approaches to promoting healthy diets adopted by governments around the world generate ethical controversy—as this chapter and this book explain. Let's begin our exploration of the ethics of healthy eating efforts by getting a handle on how public health researchers and practitioners—those who design healthy eating efforts, and often advocate for them—think about unhealthy dietary patterns.

Public health researchers have created frameworks and models of eating behaviour that identify a variety of influences on it. These include aspects related to the individual (e.g. education and taste preferences) and to the community environment; social and cultural influences; policies; and societies' basic structural features (Afshin et al. 2014; Story et al. 2008). According to many such models, frameworks, and approaches, individual eating behaviour is seen as occurring within and being influenced by local, daily food environments (e.g. retail environments, school and work environments), and these local food environments are seen as embedded within larger food systems. Various features of local food environments are identified as contributing to poor dietary quality and overconsumption, including the lower relative price of energy-dense foods (e.g. packaged foods high in calories, sugar, and sodium); the higher relative price of healthier foods such as fruits, vegetables, and whole grains; large portion sizes, which have increased over time; food marketing that makes these foods desirable and socially normative; and the sheer pervasiveness of highly palatable, energy-dense packaged food (Afshin et al. 2014; Schwartz and Brownell 2007; Story et al. 2008). Schwartz and Brownell (2007, pp. 79–80) provide a vivid description of some of these features of the food environment, framing it as a 'toxic environment':

Driving down the highway, we see dozens of drive through [sic] windows at fast food restaurants, billboards with advertisements for inexpensive snacks, and soft drinks at drugstores, and when we stop for gas, shelf after shelf of high-fat and high-sugar snacks at gas station mini marts . . . A variety of good tasting snacks and meals are now highly visible and accessible for most Americans, and there is also evidence that since the 1970s, portion sizes have gotten larger, and far exceed federal guidelines. These foods are also extremely convenient compared with home made meals, fast food and packaged foods are easier to obtain and ready to eat immediately, as they require little preparation . . . Another layer of the toxic environment that

promotes the consumption of unhealthful foods is their heavy promotion
by the food industry.

According to Schwartz and Brownell, the interaction of this 'toxic environment' with human biology and psychology creates unhealthy dietary
patterns and obesity.

Moving out from local environments, there are broader systems, policies, and social forces which are seen as shaping local food environments
and causing unhealthy dietary patterns and obesity. For example, local food
environments are embedded within larger food systems. In recent decades,
there have been changes to food systems—such as the increased processing
of food and improved food distribution—which have resulted in energy-
dense foods becoming more available. Researchers also point to other broad
social forces and trends as causes of unhealthy diet and of overweight and
obesity globally. These include rising incomes in developing countries, which
result in dietary shifts towards foods that are energy-dense and less healthy,
via what is often referred to as the 'nutrition transition' (Popkin et al. 2012);
lifestyles that do not encourage physical activity, resulting from technological advances as well as transportation and zoning policy, e.g. policies that
encourage commuting by car rather than using public transport or bicycle
(Lang and Rayner 2007); and so on.

Some researchers offer 'bigger picture' explanations for obesity, pointing
to broader economic, political, and social factors. For example, recent work
frames structural racism as a cause of higher rates of overweight, obesity,
and diet-related illness amongst some racial/ethnic groups in the US (Aaron
and Stanford 2021; Bailey et al. 2017; Bleich and Ard 2021; Dougherty et al.
2020) and identifies pathways whereby structural racism produces negative
health outcomes. For example, Bleich and Ard (2021) offer the example of
residential segregation, a manifestation of structural racism which is partly
due to a 'constellation of federal, tribal, state, and local policies as well as
private sector policies (e.g. mortgage discrimination, redlining) created in
the middle of the 20th century' (p. 234). In the US, residential segregation
persists, and affects some racial/ethnic groups in multiple ways: 'by reducing
access to quality education in childhood, which reduces economic status in
adulthood'; 'by reducing access to employment opportunities by allowing
employers to discriminate against job applicants using their neighborhood
as a deciding factor of whether the applicant would be a good employee'; and
by creating 'areas with concentrated poverty and reduced access to resources

(e.g. quality housing, healthy food, quality health care). These aggregated risks make it very hard for residents to live in healthy environments and practice healthy behaviors' (pp. 234–35).

Other explanations of rising rates of overweight and obesity point to political economy. For example, the Lancet Commission on Obesity identifies the tremendous power of the private sector as a root cause of the interrelated problems of obesity, undernutrition, and climate change (which they refer to as 'The Global Syndemic') (Swinburn et al. 2019, p. 802):

> Key aspects of the political economy have been recognized as the deep drivers that shape the very nature of the systems creating The Global Syndemic. For example, economic power has become increasingly concentrated into fewer and fewer transnational corporations, and this is certainly true in the food sector. According to the former Director General of WHO, this 'market power readily translates into political power'. Specifically, the transnational corporations lobby for fewer regulations that apply to them (eg, no regulations on marketing unhealthy food to children or warning labels on processed foods), promote regulations that apply to other sectors (eg, trade and investment agreements that bind governments to protect corporate investment interests), resist or reject taxes that apply to their products (eg, taxes on sugary drinks and energy dense, nutrient poor foods), and lobby policy makers for subsidies that benefit their businesses (eg, agricultural and transportation subsidies).

Other work also offers political economy explanations of obesity, tracing increasing rates of overweight and obesity back to neoliberalism—the political economic system that emphasizes free market capitalism and a minimal state. For example, the ideology of neoliberalism is claimed to be a cause of increasing rates of overweight and obesity: neoliberalism encourages seeing consumer choice as a right, and therefore considers the government regulation of the food marketplace illegitimate (Guthman and DuPuis 2006; Wilkerson 2010).

1.3. Healthy eating efforts

International health organizations and bodies have elevated healthy eating efforts as a global priority. This book, however, only focuses on healthy eating efforts in liberal democracies, and particularly in those that are high-income countries. Governments at all levels in these countries have enacted a range of healthy eating efforts, which take a variety of forms. To provide a sense of the range of such efforts, here are some examples, with a particular focus on the US. The efforts are organized using the NOURISHING frame-work, a helpful framework created by the World Cancer Research Fund International:

- *'Nutrition label standards and regulations on the use of claims and im-plied claims on food'*. Many countries require nutritional information to be included on food packages, and some countries also have manda-tory or voluntary front-of-package nutritional labels or warnings. These 'front-of-package' labels take different forms. In the United Kingdom, there is a 'traffic light' system that uses red, amber, or green circles to indicate the level of fat, saturated fat, sugar, or salt in food products. In the US, the Food and Drug Administration (FDA) recently redesigned the back-of-package Nutrition Facts panel, which is compulsory for all packaged foods. It is now mandatory to include a larger font size for calories, list added sugar, and use serving sizes that correspond to the servings people typically consume (FDA 2020). Also in the US, fast-food restaurants and other chain restaurants are required to post calo-ries on menus (FDA 2014).
- *'Offer healthy food and set standards in public institutions and other spe-cific settings'*. This category includes laws, institutional policies, and programmes to reduce the amount of less healthy foods and increase the availability of healthier foods in certain settings (e.g. schools, hospitals, workplaces). Several countries provide funding to schools to offer chil-dren free fruits or vegetables for snack. For example, the School Fruit and Vegetable Scheme (SFVS) in England provides a free piece of fruit or vegetable each day to children aged 4–6 who attend state-funded schools (NHS no date). In the US, several states have bans on vending machines in schools, or have restrictions on the foods that can be offered in vending machines in schools (e.g. bans on sugary drinks being offered) (Bridging the Gap 2014). This category would also include policies that leverage social support programmes to promote healthier dietary patterns. For example, public health officials and policymakers in several US states have proposed excluding sugary drinks and candy from the foods that can be purchased using food assistance provided

by the Supplemental Nutrition Assistance Programme (SNAP), which is the largest food assistance programme in the US (see Chapter 7 for an extended discussion of this policy).

- *'Use economic tools to address food affordability and purchase incentives'.* This category includes financial incentives for healthy foods as well as disincentives for some kinds of unhealthy foods.[3] An example is a tax on sugary drinks; such taxes have been implemented in several US cities and in Mexico. For example, in 2017 the city of Philadelphia adopted a 1.5 cent/ounce tax on sugary drinks and drinks with artificial sweeteners (Bleich et al. 2020). The revenue from the tax has been spent on providing public funding for early childhood education (pre-kindergarten) and on schools, parks, libraries, and recreation centres (Office of the Controller 2020).

- *'Restrict food advertising and other forms of commercial promotion'.* This category includes state regulations on food marketing as well as voluntary limitations on food marketing by companies. Examples include restrictions on the kinds of foods that can be advertised to children or bans on food marketing in schools and other children's settings.

- *'Improve nutritional quality of the whole food supply'.* This category includes bans on foods and regulations on the ingredients in foods, amongst other policies. In the US and numerous other countries, there are bans on the use of trans fat (a particularly dangerous form of fat, linked to cardiovascular disease) in packaged food. The FDA, which regulates foods, has also encouraged food companies to voluntarily adopt limits on sodium in packaged food; several other countries have mandated limits on the sodium levels in selected foods. Also included in this category are policies limiting portion sizes, including the portion sizes of packaged foods, the portions offered in fast-food restaurants, and the portions of sugary drinks. For example, as described later in more detail, in 2012 New York City (NYC) attempted to adopt a prohibition on the sale of sugary drinks larger than 16 ounces, though the policy was struck down in a court ruling and never implemented.

- *'Inform people about food and nutrition through public awareness'.* This category includes the development of national-level guidelines for a

---

[3] We use 'unhealthy foods' as shorthand to refer to foods that are widely consumed at levels that pose health risks. 'Unhealthy foods' include, e.g., candy, sugary beverages, and processed foods high in fat, sugar, or salt. 'Unhealthy foods' defined in this way is admittedly a vague category.

healthy diet. It also includes public information campaigns promoting healthy eating, e.g. campaigns promoting fruit and vegetable consumption and anti–sugary drink campaigns.

- *'Set incentives and rules to create a healthy retail and food service environment'.* This category includes efforts to increase access to healthy food (e.g. fruits, vegetables, whole grains) in neighbourhoods where access is currently limited. These efforts include programmes providing technical assistance and tax breaks for food retailers who are located in underserved areas, and for existing food retailers who increase their offerings of healthy foods. For example, an ordinance in Minneapolis, Minnesota, makes it compulsory for licensed grocery stores (including corner stores, dollar stores, gas stations, and pharmacies) to stock a minimum amount of staple foods, e.g. fruit, vegetables, and cereals (Office of Disease Prevention and Health Promotion 2020). This category also includes efforts to make healthier foods the default option; e.g. more than a dozen US cities have laws requiring restaurants to make water or milk the default drink in kids' meals, rather than sugary sodas (Center for Science in the Public Interest 2019). Another example is a law passed in the city of San Francisco, which prohibits distributing free toys with children's fast-food meals unless the meals comply with nutrition standards (Sisnowski et al. 2017).
- *'Give nutrition education and skills'.* This category includes efforts to provide nutrition education and cooking skills as well as individual-focused efforts to encourage people to change their dietary behaviour. An example would be a programme that offers women nutrition education classes, and then encourages them to adopt a dietary change for themselves and their children (e.g. filling half of their dinner plate with fruits and vegetables, as a way of increasing fruit and vegetable consumption) (Phillips-Caesar et al. 2015). Prominent in this category are school-based programmes. In the US, many healthy eating efforts are targeted at children in school or day care settings (Bennett et al. 2018). The most successful school-based programmes—e.g. the CATCH programme in the US (https://letsgo.catch.org/)—typically have multiple components, which may include one or more of the following features: nutrition and healthy eating curriculum in the classroom; take-home activities for children that reinforce in-class lessons; messaging in the school cafeteria to encourage children to eat a healthy lunch; nutritional standards for the lunches offered in the cafeteria; resources and guidance for

the cafeteria staff to help them offer and promote healthier foods; and materials for parents that reinforce the nutritional curriculum that children are learning in class, and encourage parents to eat more healthfully at home.

Many such examples of healthy eating efforts from around the world can be found in the NOURISHING database (https://www.wcrf.org/int/policy/nourishing-database).

1.4. Ethical debate about healthy eating efforts: Many participants, intellectual contexts, and agendas

The kinds of healthy eating efforts described in the previous section have generated ethical debate. This debate includes objections to these efforts as well as defences of them, and occurs in different contexts: in the popular media and on social media (Anonymous 2012a; Farley 2015); in materials produced by advocacy organizations (Food Research and Action Center [FRAC] 2017a); in legislatures, for example on the floor of the US Congress (Paarlberg et al. 2018); in the official pronouncements of government agencies and institutions (Shahin 2011); in the 'grey literature' produced by research bodies and civil society organizations (Lynch and Bassler 2014); and in academic work by a wide range of researchers, including bioethicists, political theorists, philosophers, social scientists, nutritionists, public health researchers, and a variety of other scholars who work on food systems and food studies.

Participants in the debate about healthy eating efforts contextualize this debate in broader theoretical, scientific, and policy or political contexts, and do so in different ways. They bring different agendas, methodologies, and assumptions to ethical debate about healthy eating efforts. For example, the bioethics literature includes work that critically discusses such efforts (Barnhill et al. 2014; Resnik 2010; Voigt et al. 2014). This work sometimes focuses on particular ethical arguments for and/or against specific kinds of efforts but may also take a broad ethical lens, identifying multiple kinds of ethical considerations (e.g. related to freedom, autonomy, distributive justice, health equity, etc.) that bear on healthy eating efforts (Barnhill and King 2013; ten Have et al. 2013). There is also work by philosophers, political theorists, and legal scholars (some of whom are also bioethicists) on the ethics of healthy eating efforts (Dixon 2018; Gostin 2014; Kukla 2018; Noe 2012; Williams 2015). This work fits within a larger body of work on the ethics of public health more generally (Bayer and Moreno 1986; Childress et al. 2002; Colgrove and Bayer 2005; Gostin and Gostin 2009). A central theme and preoccupation of this work is the issue of paternalism, and in particular autonomy-based objections to paternalistic public health policies. As we argue elsewhere in this book, this emphasis on paternalism may have occluded other important ethical issues with healthy eating policy, including those concerning its legitimacy and justifiability.

There is also a significant body of work by public health researchers and practitioners that ethically appraises healthy eating policy; some of this work is produced by interdisciplinary teams including both public health experts and ethicists (Grummon et al. 2020; Kass et al. 2014; Rajagopal et al. 2018; ten Have et al. 2013). In some cases, this work explicitly identifies itself as ethical analysis (Grummon et al. 2020). In other cases, ethical assumptions may be made or ethical conclusions reached, even if the work does not explicitly identify itself as ethics (Roberto et al. 2015). While some work by public health researchers and practitioners considers the ethics of healthy eating efforts in an open-ended or critical way (Grummon et al. 2020), other work is unabashed advocacy for healthy eating efforts (Brownell et al. 2010; Farley 2015).

Some work by public health experts that advocates for healthy eating efforts frames these efforts as justifiable responses to an industry—the food and beverage industry—that pervasively influences consumers in problematic (i.e. manipulative, exploitative, and deceptive) ways (Farley 2015; Frieden 2013; Nestle and Ludwig 2010; Roberto et al. 2015) and that works behind the scenes to shape public opinion and public policy to its advantage (Aaron and Siegel 2016; Brownell and Warner 2009; Nestle 2007). In other words, healthy eating efforts are justified by situating them within a particular broader context: there is an unethical and harmful industry with significant power over consumers, and healthy eating efforts are needed to counteract this power. Some work draws parallels between the food industry and the tobacco industry (Brownell and Warner 2009; Nestle 2007), arguing that the food industry uses some of the same tactics that the tobacco industry employed to distort science, deceive the public, and stifle government regulation. This situates healthy eating efforts in the historical context of relatively aggressive public health efforts against tobacco use and the tobacco industry.

There is a body of critical work on healthy eating efforts and obesity discourse by scholars from multiple academic disciplines (e.g. critical race and gender studies, disability studies, geography, sociology, philosophy). This work may make ethical claims, or assume certain ethical claims, even if it does not explicitly identify itself as ethics. A theme of some critical work is that our discourse about obesity needs to be understood in its cultural context, as reflecting moral attitudes, ideologies, and cultural norms about eating, fat, pleasure, body shape, disability, race, and gender (Aphramor 2009; Kukla 2018; Sanders 2019; Wilkerson 2010; Womack 2014), even if on its surface this discourse is about identifying and addressing a public health problem.

Some critical work contextualizes debates about healthy eating efforts within broader debates about the role of the state in promoting health and debates about personal responsibility and health (Guthman 2011; Kirkland 2011). For example, healthy eating efforts that aim to produce individual behaviour change (e.g. food labelling, nutrition education) are seen as reflecting healthism—the moralization of health, such that health becomes a 'super value' and good citizenship requires good health (Guthman 2011, pp. 52–53, 55; Mayes and Thompson 2014). They are also seen as reflecting 'responsibilization', i.e. 'the notion that each individual must act to take care of herself so that she does not become a burden on society—by smoking, by failing to be careful during pregnancy, or by getting fat, for example' (Kirkland 2011, pp. 466–67). Responsibilization is seen as assigning responsibility to individuals for problems that are actually social and environmental in origin, and thus should be addressed through collective solutions rather than efforts at individual behaviour change. For some such critiques of healthy eating policy, healthism and responsibilization are seen, in turn, as manifestations of neoliberalism and of neoliberal ideology, which emphasize individual responsibility for behaviour rather than collective responsibility and collective solutions (Guthman 2011; Guthman and DuPuis 2006). Thus the broader intellectual and political context for some critiques of healthy eating efforts is a critique of neoliberalism and of its social and political manifestations.

Lastly, there are a range of perspectives on healthy eating efforts offered by different kinds of advocates and advocacy movements. For example, the food justice movement—a social justice movement that addresses a range of problems in the food system—has identified increasing access to healthy and culturally appropriate food as a central goal (see e.g. FoodPrint 2021).

Inadequate access to healthy food is contextualized as a form of injustice, and often as a form of racial injustice (Alkon and Agyeman 2011). Other advocates have brought a critical perspective to healthy eating efforts. For example, some anti-hunger advocates in the US have objected to efforts to exclude sugary drinks and candy from food assistance programmes (FRAC 2017a), arguing that these efforts single out low-income people for restriction and control (FRAC 2017a; Paarlberg et al. 2018). This criticism echoes a long-standing critique that public assistance programmes micromanage the choices and lives of low-income people in a disrespectful, demeaning, and unjust way. Schwartz (2017, p. S203) aptly describes the broader orientation that anti-hunger advocates bring to this issue and that grounds their critique: '[i]f the fundamental mission of your work is to protect the basic rights and dignity of people living in poverty, it makes sense that you would not agree with any policy that exerted control over how some citizens spend their money just because they are poor'. In other words, anti-hunger advocates contextualize healthy eating efforts within a broader political context, one in which their role is to advocate that more resources, more choice, and more dignity should be afforded to low-income people.

As this discussion has hopefully made clear, a wide range of scholars, researchers, and practitioners engage with healthy eating efforts. They situate such efforts within different, broader contexts—theoretical, historical, and political. Depending on how healthy eating efforts are contextualized, different broad ethical perspectives on such efforts may emerge, be salient, and appear justifiable. For example, seeing healthy eating efforts as analogous to (favourably assessed) anti-tobacco efforts suggests that they are necessary and justifiable, whereas viewing healthy eating efforts in the context of 'responsibilization' and healthism suggests that these efforts are ethically problematic because they inappropriately pin responsibility for eating and health on individuals.

We cannot do justice here to this large, sprawling, critical discussion of healthy eating efforts. Instead, we distil from it four areas of ethical concern with healthy eating efforts, which we discuss in section 1.6.

1.5. Healthy *and* sustainable diets

Before turning to our discussion of the ethical concerns raised by healthy eating efforts, we would like to briefly consider another important ethical perspective on such efforts. According to this perspective, overweight and obesity are one negative effect associated with our dietary patterns amongst other morally important negative effects. For example, work on the 'triple burden of malnutrition' identifies obesity as one of three forms of malnutrition, along with undernutrition (not consuming enough food) and micronutrient deficiencies. All three forms of malnutrition are common globally (Béné et al. 2020, p. 2):

Molnutrogenic

> At present, more than 820 million people remain undernourished, 149 million children are stunted, and 49.5 million are wasted. While the precise figures are uncertain, there are an estimated 2 billion people with micronutrient deficiencies and 2.1 billion adults overweight or obese. Overall, 'unhealthy' diets are estimated to be the most significant risk factor for global burden of disease in the world. Simultaneously, food systems are recognized to be one of the largest causes of global environmental changes, leading to soil degradation, deforestation, and depletion of freshwater resources. Recent estimates show that food production is responsible for 19 to 29% of global greenhouse gas emissions.

As this passage makes it clear, our dietary patterns are a problem not only because they result in multiple forms of malnutrition that have bad health effects but also because of the environmental impacts of food production. Some dietary patterns have a much higher average environmental footprint than others, because some foods take significantly more land, water, chemical inputs (e.g. fertilizer), or energy to produce and/or are associated with higher greenhouse gas emissions or other forms of pollution. In particular, production of animal-source foods is generally associated with higher environmental impacts than plant-based foods, and thus dietary patterns higher in animal-source foods have a higher-than-average environmental footprint (Ranganathan et al. 2016).

The food system already accounts for around a quarter of total greenhouse gas emissions (Poore and Nemecek 2018), and food production is 'the largest cause of global environmental change' (Willett et al. 2019, p. 3) using 40% of global land and 70% of total freshwater (Springmann et al. 2018; Willett et al. 2019). As the world population grows, food demand will increase, perhaps by as much as 50 to 60% by 2050. As more societies around the globe rise out of poverty, their members will have more money to spend on food and will eat more meat, if the past is any guide. As a result, the environmental impacts of the food system are on pace to increase significantly, perhaps by 50 to 90% by 2050 (Springmann et al. 2018). As a result, it will be a major challenge to meet overall goals for reductions in greenhouse gas emissions and to keep the food system within other safe environmental limits (Willett et al. 2019).

Some influential scientific work concludes that keeping the food system within safe environmental limits, while producing enough food to feed a growing population, will require three changes: first, widespread adoption of more sustainable agricultural production practises; second, significant reductions in how much food is wasted, so that less food production will be needed to meet food demand; and third, shifts towards plant-based diets, which have smaller average environmental footprints. In support of this third change, some scientific work aims to identify dietary patterns that are environmentally sustainable and also healthy. For example, the EAT-Lancet commission (Willett et al. 2019) constructed a 'planetary diet'—a diet designed to allow for optimal human health, and which could be produced for 10 billion people in 2050 while keeping the food system within proposed environmental limits. As compared to the average diet in high-income countries, this diet includes dramatically less animal-source food consumption; e.g. it includes about one serving of beef per week, which would amount to about an 80% decrease in per capita beef consumption in the US.

The upshot of scientific work on sustainable diets is that dietary patterns should shift dramatically towards more sustainable diets (e.g. plant-based diets), amongst other changes. This has ethical implications for healthy eating policy. Efforts to shift dietary patterns should be mindful of two broad goals: shifting dietary patterns in *both* healthier *and* more sustainable directions. If these goals are not harmonized, efforts to promote more sustainable dietary patterns could end up having negative effects on health, or vice versa. For example, some plant-based diets are not optimal for health (e.g. diets high in starches and grains, especially in processed form), and thus the promotion of plant-based diets without regard for the health effects of these diets may not produce optimal health outcomes. As Fanzo (2019, p. 167) writes:

> There are diets that can be either environmentally sustainable and not healthy, or healthy and not environmentally sustainable . . . For example, diets with low dietary diversity and which derive the majority of dietary energy from starches and grains, have lower environmental footprints. These low-impact diets often fail to address individuals' micro- and macronutrient

needs . . . They can also be associated with high levels of sugar and salt consumption . . . and low levels of key micronutrients, such as iron and zinc.

Just as not all environmentally sustainable dietary patterns are healthy, not all healthy dietary patterns could be widely adopted in an environmentally sustainable way. For example, US dietary recommendations advise consuming more fish; if these recommendations were widely followed, this could deplete global fish supplies and threaten fishers' livelihoods (IOM and NRC 2015). Thus governments keen to promote healthier dietary patterns should consider pursuing both goals simultaneously, through efforts that identify and promote dietary patterns that are both sustainable and healthy.

1.6. Ethical concerns with healthy eating efforts

This section briefly lays out four areas of ethical concern with healthy eating efforts (Barnhill 2019): concerns with the limited effectiveness of healthy eating efforts; ethical concerns with choice, liberty, and freedom; ethical concerns related to equity, fairness, and justice; and ethical concerns related to stigma, responsibility, and moral blame.

1.6.1. Concerns with the limited effectiveness of healthy eating efforts

Some researchers and advocates argue that certain kinds of healthy eating efforts, namely individual-focused efforts such as nutrition education or dietary change interventions, have limited effectiveness, and therefore that these individual-focused efforts are insufficient and need to be complemented or replaced with interventions that are focused on changing food environments (Roberto et al. 2015; Schwartz and Brownell 2007; Story et al. 2008). Some scholars go further, arguing that obesity prevention efforts in general have limited effectiveness. These scholars claim that the focus of public policy should be on interventions aimed at addressing broader social and economic factors that influence health and which can accomplish multiple goals at the same time, *not* policies that only focus on obesity prevention per se (Williams 2015). For example, Williams (2015) highlights the mixed and discouraging evidence regarding community-level obesity prevention efforts. He argues that the focus of public policy should *not* be on the wider implementation of community-level obesity prevention efforts but instead on broader social and economic factors that influence health. Julie Guthman and Anna Kirkland also call for policymakers to shift their focus from efforts to alter the food environment to broader social policies, e.g. policies increasing access to healthcare and transportation (Guthman 2011; Kirkland 2011).

Despite these critical voices, expert recommendations continue to emphasize the importance of changing dietary patterns directly, and of adopting policy measures squarely aimed at this goal (Barnhill et al. 2018; CFS 2021; IOM and CAPOP 2012; Swinburn et al. 2019).

1.6.2. Concerns with choice, liberty, freedom, and paternalism

As discussed earlier, the healthy eating efforts recommended by public health authorities include increased regulation of the food industry—reformulating products, banning ingredients, placing limits on portion size, taxing products, and restricting food marketing. Such policies generate pushback and ethical discussion concerned with choice, liberty, freedom, and paternalism.

For example, a notorious example of a choice-limiting healthy eating effort is the failed NYC soda ban. In 2012, former NYC mayor Michael Bloomberg proposed, and then the NYC Board of Health adopted, a prohibition on the sale of sugary drinks larger than 16 ounces in some food retailers. The policy was intended to reduce consumption of sugary drinks and thereby reduce rates of diet-related illness. It was meant to go into effect in March 2013 but was struck down in a court ruling and was never implemented.

After proposing the soda ban, Mayor Bloomberg was pilloried as 'nannying'. In 2012, the Center for Consumer Freedom (an industry-funded group) took out a full-page ad in the *New York Times* showing him dressed as a nanny (Dicker 2012). 'Nanny Bloomberg has taken his strange obsession with what you eat one step further', the ad read. 'New Yorkers need a Mayor, not a Nanny' (Dicker 2012). Even the *New York Times*, a left-leaning paper and one generally favourably disposed towards public health, referred to the soda ban as 'nannying' in an editorial entitled 'A Soda Ban Too Far' (Anonymous 2012a).

Defenders of healthy eating efforts sometimes respond to such charges of 'nannying' by reframing these efforts: healthy eating efforts, they claim, do not patronizingly protect consumers from themselves, as the nannying charge implies, but rather protect consumers from a food industry that undermines their autonomy by misleading, deceiving, manipulating, or exploiting them (Farley 2015; Frieden 2013; Moss 2013; Nestle and Ludwig 2010; Roberto et al. 2015). Opposition to healthy eating efforts is sometimes explained as partially a product of the food industry working behind the scenes to shape public opinion (Brownell and Warner 2009; Nestle 2007). However, our perspective is that public resistance to 'nannying' healthy eating efforts should not be seen as just the result of food industry machinations. As we discuss at greater length in Chapter 4, there are long-standing philosophical objections to government paternalism, and the 'nannying' charge may be a way of registering these kinds of objections.

Government paternalism—i.e. government efforts that aim to make the individual better off and are motivated by a negative judgement about the individual's ability to advance her own welfare and/or interfere with their freedom without their consent (Dworkin 2020; Quong 2011)—has been objected to as degrading, demeaning, and failing to treat people as equals (Conly 2013a), and as simply counterproductive: individuals know better than the government how to promote their own welfare, and therefore governments' interference with individuals' own efforts will only gum up the works and make those individuals worse off. Paternalistic public health efforts, in particular, have been objected to as incorrectly assuming that people value health more than they actually do (Noe 2013; Pugh 2014). Paternalistic policies that limit choice have also been objected to as violating individual autonomy (Dworkin 1972; Feinberg 1986; Mill 2006), though some theorists have defended paternalism, even when it violates autonomy. For example, Sarah Conly (2013a, 2013b) argues that paternalistic policies that prevent irrational eating, e.g. imposing limits on portion sizes in restaurants, can be ethically justifiable even though they violate autonomy; such policies, Conly argues, respect individuals by helping them achieve their long-term goals of staying healthy and living a long life. Another response to the charge of paternalism is to argue that healthy eating efforts should not even be considered *paternalistic*, since their ultimate goal is not to increase individual welfare but to reduce the costs of poor health for society and thus advance the common good (Bayer and Moreno 1986; Gostin and Gostin 2009). This set of ethical concerns is discussed in more detail in Chapter 3.

1.6.3. Concerns with equity, fairness, and justice

Another set of ethical arguments surrounding healthy eating efforts centres on justice, equity, and fairness.

On the one hand, some might argue that justice demands healthy eating efforts. For example, ensuring equality of opportunity for all may require healthy eating efforts that help to maintain good health broadly throughout society. In addition, responding adequately to structural injustice, e.g. structural racism, may require recognizing the many ways in which structural injustice shapes people's dietary patterns and undermines their health, and working to remedy this.

Along with arguments that justice demands healthy eating efforts in general, there are justice-based arguments for specific kinds of healthy eating efforts. For example, lack of access to healthy food in some neighbourhoods is often seen as unjust: as a matter of justice, people are entitled to access to healthy, culturally appropriate food. Furthermore, there is a distinct, racial justice argument for increasing food access: disparities in food access reflect specific historical injustices as past housing discrimination in the US (a form of institutional racism) has resulted in Black Americans disproportionately living in areas with poor access to healthy food (Braveman et al. 2011; Kumanyika 2005). Thus, there are multiple distinct justice-based arguments for efforts to increase access to healthy food. Indeed, increasing access to healthy, culturally appropriate food is a goal of the 'food justice' movement (Alkon 2011; Morales 2011).

On the other hand, there are justice- and fairness-based arguments *against* some kinds of healthy eating efforts. For example, financial disincentives, such as taxes on sugary drinks, are criticized for being regressive (i.e. they absorb a larger share of the income of low-income people) and, for that reason, unfair or inequitable. In response, others claim that disadvantaged groups are in fact the most likely to benefit from taxes on sugary drinks, because these groups generally display higher rates of obesity; therefore, far from being regressive and unfair, these efforts can actually disproportionately *benefit* disadvantaged groups (Barry et al. 2013). Another example of justice- and fairness-based objections to healthy eating efforts concerns efforts in the US to exclude sugary drinks and candy from the foods eligible for purchase with food assistance. These efforts have been objected to as unfair, i.e. as unfairly targeting low-income groups in ways that may not be welcomed by them and that smack of 'micro-managing' their personal choices (Barnhill and King 2013).

1.6.4. Concerns with stigma, responsibility, and moral blame

Another set of concerns with healthy eating efforts centre on stigma, responsibility, and moral blame (Womack 2014). The public discourse about overweight and obesity has been critiqued as pervaded with negative moral judgements of people who are overweight, e.g. that they are lazy or lack self-control (Puhl and Heuer 2010), and as feeding into and contributing to stigmatization of and discrimination against people who are overweight and obese.

Obesity discourse in general, along with some specific healthy eating efforts, has been critiqued as stigmatizing. For example, some public information campaigns that present people who are overweight, or parents of children who are overweight, in a negative light have been critiqued as stigmatizing, as have some campaigns that seem designed to cause guilt, shame, scorn, and other negative emotions (Abu-Odeh 2014; Fairchild et al. 2015; Kliff 2012). Stigmatization of overweight and obesity is objected to on ethical but also practical grounds: some researchers argue that stigmatization is counterproductive, because it reduces the utilization of healthcare by people who are overweight, reduces the quality of care provided to them, and increases stress and unhealthy diet (Goldberg and Puhl 2013; Puhl and Heuer 2010). It is worth noting that there may be significant variability in what is meant by 'stigma' and in the charge that healthy eating efforts are stigmatizing. 'Stigma' and 'stigmatization' are sometimes used to refer to a severe and all-encompassing form of social sanction that involves a loss of status, shame, and self-punishment, but are also used more loosely to refer to public disapproval, self-directed shame, social marginalization, and other related phenomena (Bayer 2008a, 2008b; Burris 2008).

Sanders (2019) argues that fat stigma has fused with negative racial stereotypes in obesity discourse in the US. Despite the fact that there are high rates of obesity across demographic groups, obesity has been linked with race and gender—e.g. Black women are often presented as the 'face' of obesity, and in this way obesity is racialized. Furthermore,

> because they unfold in a political context pervaded by negative stereotypes of black women . . . discourses that racialize obesity tend to reproduce these stereotypes . . . By personifying the typical obese American as black and female and by invoking tropes of black women as indulgent, undisciplined bad mothers who exploit state funds and deplete the economy, even

well-meaning and left-leaning raced and gendered anti-obesity discourses invite and justify the systematic practices of discrimination and exclusion that sustain status quo racial inequality. (p. 290)

Thus, on Sanders' critique, fat stigma is a kind of force multiplier of the stigmatization of Black women.

Another theme in critical work is that the public discourse about obesity and diet involves attributing responsibility and moral blame to people who are overweight for being overweight, when these attributions may be inappropriate because overweight has environmental, social, and structural causes and thus is not something individuals should be morally blamed for (see Brownell et al. 2010; Guthman 2011, Kirkland 2011, and Dixon 2018 for discussion of obesity and responsibility).

1.7. The place of food and eating in daily life and life plans

The (familiar) ethical concerns discussed in the previous section are important but not exhaustive. There is another critical angle on healthy eating that has not been sufficiently emphasized, either in the design of healthy eating efforts or in their ethical critique. This critical angle starts with the appreciation of eating as a lived experience that plays various roles, positive and negative, in the lives of individuals, families, and communities (Barnhill et al. 2014; Mayes and Thompson 2014; Mulvaney-Day and Womack 2009). What people eat often represents their best effort to navigate dilemmas surrounding food (e.g. do I feed my children a healthier meal or a meal that I can make quickly at the end of a long day?) and to manage the trade-offs inherent to food and eating. In the following pages we introduce this critical perspective on eating and consider some of the issues it raises.

1.7.1. The instrumental and intrinsic value of food and eating

Food is a resource necessary for sustenance and survival, and, as healthy eating efforts emphasize, food is a potential source of good (or bad) nutrition and health. But in addition to its role in promoting nutrition and physical health, food serves other personal and social functions (Barnhill et al. 2014; Mayes and Thompson 2014; Mulvaney-Day and Womack 2009). Food and eating can provide pleasure, comfort, satiation, and other positive experiences. They can also serve social functions (Counihan and Van Esterik 2013), since food is central to virtually all kinds of human relationships and social groups. Eating together, sharing food, and having a common cuisine contribute to building and fostering social relationships within families, between friends and colleagues, and within larger social groups (Mulvaney-Day and Womack 2009). Preparing food for someone is a way of expressing love. Social relationships can also help to increase our food resources, as when people borrow food from one another in times of need, thus reducing food insecurity (Mulvaney-Day and Womack 2009). In short, shared food experiences create, express, and reinforce social bonds.

Food is also linked to social and cultural identities. Social and cultural groups often have distinctive patterns of eating and foods that are assigned special significance (Anderson 2005; Counihan and Van Esterik 2013; Guptill et al. 2013, Chap. 2; Rozin and Siegal 2003). Food practises are one way in which we construct personal identities and group identities, and are a powerful way to communicate our identities to others: '[w]hat foods we eat, how and when we prepare, serve, and consume them, are all types of identity work—activity through which we define for ourselves and others who we are socially and culturally' (Guptill et al. 2013, p. 18). Part of identifying as Italian or Japanese for many people is appreciating traditional or distinctive Italian or Japanese foods. Food is used to celebrate special occasions in ways that are often culturally distinctive as well as socially and personally valuable. Often it is less healthy foods that are used to mark special occasions: in the US, e.g., these might include birthday cupcakes, wedding cakes, Halloween candies, and Valentine's chocolates. Food is also linked to religious identity; religions can prescribe patterns of eating, including special foods as part of rituals, special foods on holidays, periodic fasting and abstinence, as well as standing prohibitions of certain foods.

Food also has aesthetic value and can be central to a person's self-expression and creativity, or to their aesthetic appreciation of a certain place. Furthermore, food can be central to the expression and fulfilment of certain moral and ethical commitments, as in the case of food choices driven by an ethical commitment to animal rights and welfare, human rights, environmental justice, or global justice (De Tavernier 2012).

Thus, food and eating can be instrumental to various ends, including survival, nutrition, short-term physical well-being (e.g. having energy), long-term health, and longevity, and social ends such as forming and strengthening relationships, creating and expressing individual and group identity, and living out one's religious or moral commitments. Moreover, food and eating can cause positive subjective experiences (e.g. pleasure, comfort, stress relief, satiation), and these positive subjective experiences can have psychological benefits.

Along with instrumental value, eating and food experiences can have intrinsic value. For example, eating can be a positive subjective experience (e.g. pleasurable, comforting) that is intrinsically valuable. Eating and food experiences can also have aesthetic value, and in that sense be intrinsically valuable. Furthermore, food experiences can have expressive value, expressing emotions (e.g. love for the person you are making food for), moral values, and personal identity (including religious, cultural, ethnic, national, regional, and gender identities), and in that way also have intrinsic value.

1.7.2. Trade-offs and dilemmas

Just as food experiences can be instrumental to achieving our ends (e.g. the end of living a long, healthy life, or the end of having close loving relationships within our family), so too food experiences can undermine the achievement of our ends. Food and eating can be a source of health risks and poor health; if one of our goals is maintaining good health and living a long life, unhealthy dietary patterns can undermine the achievement of this end. Food and eating can also have significant economic and practical costs, in terms of money, time, effort, and attention; incurring such costs can undermine the achievement of other ends (one example, which we will discuss later, involves mothers reporting that making a home-cooked meal at the end of a busy day takes time away from helping their children with their homework).

Just as eating and food experiences can have instrumental disvalue, so too can they have *intrinsic* disvalue. For example, eating can be disgusting or a source of displeasure, rather than pleasurable, comforting, or aesthetically pleasing. Eating certain foods can be misaligned with our moral values and social identities, and can have intrinsic disvalue in that way.

Because food and eating have so many different kinds of value and disvalue, there can be conflicts and trade-offs. Consider this hypothetical example:

Every Sunday after church, a family attends the weekly potluck supper, at which a variety of unhealthy but delicious foods is always served. The parents know the supper is unhealthy and they would like their family to eat more healthfully, but they attend the church supper because they're not willing to miss out on seeing their friends, staying up to date on what's happening in the church, and making sure their children feel like part of the church community. Also, attending the church supper was important to them growing up and is a tradition that they value and would like to pass on to their children. (Barnhill et al. 2014, p. 197)

The parents decide to attend the church supper, even though they want their family to eat more healthfully, because for them it is a significant experience which is valuable for many different reasons: it is enjoyable, it strengthens social bonds, and it is a meaningful tradition that they are keen to transmit to their children.

In sum, eating unhealthfully can have various kinds of value; eating healthfully can have different kinds of disvalue; and thus, adopting a healthier dietary pattern can involve trade-offs between valued experiences and valued ends.

There is some (but surprisingly little) qualitative research by social scientists that captures the trade-offs at play with healthy eating. For example, Bowen et al. (2014) examined mothers' experiences making home-cooked meals; they interviewed 150 Black, white, and Latina mothers of different income levels in the US, and carried out in-home observations. They were interested in home-cooked meals because the recommendation to cook meals at home—rather than eating in restaurants or eating packaged, processed foods—is a mainstay in healthy eating advice. They found that some mothers face basic economic constraints: they do not have kitchens or basic cooking equipment (e.g. knives). Time was also a major issue: some mothers, especially lower-income mothers, did not have predictable work schedules, and this made planning ahead and cooking difficult for them. Furthermore, some mothers of middle-class background did have access to adequate kitchens and jobs with predictable schedules but still experienced time constraints: their kids were clamouring for attention while they were trying to cook dinner, and realistically they had to choose between cooking and spending time with their children. Other research has also found that there may be higher time costs associated with healthy food preparation (Jabs et al. 2007; Monsivais et al. 2014), and thus opportunity costs associated with healthy eating (Cawley and Liu 2012). Working mothers report trading off food preparation and mealtime so that their children will have more time for homework and get to bed on time (Devine et al. 2006).

Bowen et al. (2014, p. 25) also found that mothers experienced significant stress and frustration about cooking falling short of their expectations and goals:

> [One mother] explained, 'When we get home it's such a rush. I just don't know what happens to the time. I am so frustrated. That's why I get so angry! I get frustrated 'cause I'm like, I wanna make this good meal that's really healthy and I like to cook 'cause it's kind of my way to show them that I love them, "This is my love for you guys!" And then I wind up at the end just, you know, grrr! Mad at the food because it takes me so long . . .' Even the extensive prep work that Elaine did on the weekends didn't translate into a relaxing meal during the weekday. Instead, like so many mothers, Elaine felt frustrated and inadequate about not living up to the ideal home-cooked meals.

Another notable finding from Bowen et al. is that making and serving healthy home-cooked meals brought on interpersonal conflict:

> 'I don't need it. I don't want it. I never had it', exclaimed 4-year-old Rashan when his mom served him an unfamiliar side dish. Rashan's reaction was not uncommon. We rarely observed a meal in which at least one family member didn't complain about the food they were served. Some mothers coaxed their children to eat by playing elaborate games or by hand-feeding them. (p. 24)

Parents frequently report making dietary trade-offs to keep the peace and avoid conflict at mealtime (Bowen and Devine 2011). All in all, Bowen et al.'s (2014) study and related research find that making healthy, home-cooked meals involves a series of trade-offs and negative effects for the US mothers they studied.

The work of sociologist Priya Fielding-Singh also provides insight into the lived experience of healthy eating in families. Fielding-Singh interviewed 160 parents and adolescents of different income levels in the US, and observed families. She found that adolescents of all income levels pestered their parents to have junk food, but that there was a sharp difference between affluent and low-income parents in how they responded: while '96 percent of the affluent families in [her] sample reported that they regularly denied their adolescents' junk food requests for health reasons, just 13% of low-income families said the same' (Fielding-Singh 2017). Fielding-Singh found that allowing children to have junk food had different meanings for parents of different income levels:

> For low-income parents, daily life in poverty stripped them of opportunities to say 'yes' to their adolescents' requests, be it a new pair of shoes or a trip to Disneyland. Food could be an important exception: low-SES [socio-economic status] parents often had enough money to oblige adolescents' inexpensive food requests. A bag of Cheetos was almost always within financial reach. Thus, parents obliged adolescents' wishes to compensate for scarcity in other domains. Doing so not only emotionally satisfied their children; critically, it also gave parents a sense of worth and competence as caregivers in a context where those feelings were constantly in jeopardy. Among affluent parents, food took on a different, but similarly potent, meaning. These parents derived a sense of worth as caregivers in curtailing—rather than obliging—adolescents' unhealthy dietary desires. Raising their adolescents in contexts of abundance, food offered these parents an ongoing medium for teaching restraint and delayed gratification . . . Within these vastly different contexts, food takes on vastly different meanings. The poor parents I spoke with said 'yes' to their kids out of a deep desire to care and provide for them amidst constrained material circumstances, not out of disregard or a devaluation of their health. Similarly, the affluent parents I met denied their adolescents' food requests in an earnest effort to instill in them healthy lifelong habits, not to deprive them. (Fielding-Singh 2017; see also Fielding-Singh 2018)

Fielding-Singh's work provides a poignant example of the value of consumption of unhealthy foods, both instrumental and intrinsic: letting their children eat junk food has positive intrinsic value to the low-income parents Fielding-Singh studied, as a way of saying yes to them, demonstrating care, and shoring up their self-conception as parents. For these parents, consistently saying no to their adolescents' junk food requests could involve interpersonal and psychological costs.

The work of Bowen et al. and Fielding-Singh identifies economic (time, money, effort), interpersonal, and psychological-emotional costs for families of cooking and eating healthfully. Other qualitative research and anecdotal evidence also identify economic, social, and psychological costs of dietary change, both for parents and for people more generally (Devine and Barnhill 2018). Efforts to eat more healthfully can put strain on social relationships. People adopting healthier dietary patterns have reported that their dietary changes can create tension at mealtimes, e.g. because family members who prepare food feel slighted (Bowen and Devine 2011) or because those trying to eat more healthfully are nagged for not following through (Rosland et al. 2010) or when family food preparers change the rules for family meals and expect others to go along (Eldridge et al. 2016). Those adopting healthier dietary patterns report no longer feeling comfortable attending community events or work events involving food, or meals with extended family, because their food choices set them off as different (Devine and Barnhill 2018). Thus it appears that there are trade-offs between common forms of socializing and adopting healthier dietary patterns.

Efforts to eat more healthfully—especially when they are not successful—can also have psychological costs, including discouragement, self-blame, and loss of self-efficacy and self-esteem (Devine and Barnhill 2018; Linde et al. 2006). Adopting healthier dietary patterns may have other sorts of psychological costs too. For example, consider this quote from a participant in a weight loss programme: '[e]ating stops the process of my brain going. It offers relief from thoughts that might actually be quite uncomfortable' (Byrne et al. 2003, p. 960). When eating certain foods provides comfort or is a coping strategy, reducing or eliminating consumption of those foods will have some psychological costs.

What this research shows is that there are trade-offs involved in adopting healthier dietary patterns. This means that people may experience dilemmas surrounding healthy eating: people may have a range of ends to which eating is relevant, and they may not be able to simultaneously realize all those ends. For example, a parent may have a range of ends, including her children being healthy, her children feeling loved, the family spending quality time together at mealtime, and maintaining a positive self-conception and resilience as a parent. But given the context of her life—time scarcity, money scarcity, her children's desires to eat junk food, all of which are influenced by the broader social and economic context—she may not be able to simultaneously realize all these ends. Some ends may have to be sacrificed so that other ends can be achieved. For some parents, the best way to navigate this dilemma may be to pursue healthy eating and deal with the trade-offs: spending more money on healthier food, denying the kids' requests for junk food, spending less time with the kids in the evening in order to cook a healthy dinner, and weathering the interpersonal conflict at mealtime that comes from feeding the kids a healthier meal they do not want. For other parents, the best way to navigate this dilemma may be to de-emphasize health and healthy eating. Which trade-offs are the best ones for someone to make depends, in large part, upon what their ends are, how these ends fit into their life plan, and how these ends align with their conception of the good. In the next section we present a theoretical framework for thinking about healthy eating: people have *ends*, and these ends are nestled within *life plans*, and these ends and life plans may (or may not) cohere with people's *conception of the good*.

1.7.3. *The place of food and eating in life plans*

People make choices, engage in actions, have experiences. Sometimes these choices, actions, and experiences further the person's chosen ends, and sometimes they do not. For example, a mother's choice to give in to her children's junk food requests may further her end of making her children feel loved. We can see specific ends as nestled within *life plans*, which are longer-term, stable, structured plans for a life. For example, a mother's end of making her children feel loved may be part of a life plan that includes maintaining close, loving relationships with her children throughout her life. Life plans are sometimes articulated, made explicit, and endorsed, but sometimes remain implicit and unarticulated.

Another element of our theoretical framework is the idea of a *conception of the good*, i.e. 'an ordered family of final ends and aims which specifies a person's conception of what is of value in human life or, alternatively, of what is regarded as a fully worthwhile life' (Rawls 2001, p. 19). Conceptions of the good are sometimes explicitly articulated or fashioned and explicitly endorsed. But conceptions of the good may also be adopted and lived out even without being explicitly articulated or endorsed; e.g. some people may be socialized into cultural or religious practises which give value to their lives while not being the object of explicit endorsement or critical reflection (e.g. Parekh 2006). Life plans sometimes fit well with a person's *conception of the good*, but there can also be misalignment between a person's life plan and her conception of the good. For example, suppose that someone's conception of the good life is a life full of close friendships and family relationships, and a long life that includes having grandchildren and watching them grow up. However, suppose that that person is pursuing a life plan that de-emphasizes personal relationships in favour of working very long hours and optimizing career success, and which de-emphasizes preserving health in favour of convenience and immediate pleasure (such that, e.g., she does not spend time exercising and does not pay attention to eating healthfully). The life plan that she is pursuing, day to day, is at odds with her conception of the good life.

Food-related experiences can be central to people's life plans.[4] In some cases, specific food-related experiences are a central constitutive part of one's chosen life plan. For example, if someone's life plan is to open a restaurant and be a chef, her life plan will include a number of food-related experiences (aesthetic, social, etc.) that are directly central to it.[5] In other cases, certain kinds of food experiences may be *indirectly central* to someone's life plan, because these food experiences are central to something else that is central to her life plan. For example, central to a person's life plan might be a rich family life which involves sharing food experiences amongst other things or the expression of a cultural or ethnic identity that is experienced with others via food and eating or aesthetic experiences that involve food (e.g. regularly experiencing new foods or becoming an expert on haute cuisine). In these examples, there are personal, family, social/community, or cultural dimensions that are central to a person's life plan, and food experiences that are central to those dimensions.

Another connection between food experiences and life plans is that certain kinds of food experiences may be a practical *necessity* for one's life plan while not being central to it (directly or indirectly). For example, being able to access affordable, nutritious food may be necessary for a person's ability to be healthy and therefore to pursue a life plan that requires good health, even if their life plan does not centrally involve eating nutritious food. Some level of access to convenient food could also be necessary for some people's ability to pursue their life plans (whatever these are), given the significant time and

---

[4] See Mayes and Thompson (2014, p. 166) for a related discussion. They argue that 'food choices and culinary practices present a rich diversity of avenues for humans to experiment with in order to creatively enrich and cultivate a good life'.

[5] It should be noted here that not all those food experiences that are central to one's life plans are also valuable. For example, if you run a restaurant because being a chef and/or restaurateur is your life plan, central to that life plan will be complying with the required food hygiene regulations, attending the required food hygiene training courses, learning how to handle food, etc. (since failing to comply with these requirements could lead to the end of your life plan), yet you probably would not consider those food-related experiences valuable per se.

effort costs that can be associated with cooking and eating. For example, suppose that someone's life plan includes a demanding career that requires working long hours. That person will not be able to spend much time procuring food or cooking, and thus convenience vis-à-vis food will be necessary to enable her life plan.

1.7.4. Unhealthy dietary patterns

The upshot of the previous sections is that instances of eating unhealthy foods—and even an overall dietary pattern that significantly increases health risks—can be someone's way of dealing with the trade-offs inherent to healthy eating in the context of her life. Unhealthy dietary patterns can represent someone making the best of the dilemmas she faces. Moreover, they may be consistent with someone's life plans and conception of the good.

But it is also important to recognize that people's life plans are complex, and people may struggle to find coherence between different strands of their life plans. There can be tensions, often unworked out, within life plans. For example, someone's life plan may include being successful at their chosen career (which may require working very long hours) *and* living a long life (which requires eating healthfully and getting a decent amount of physical activity) *and* raising healthy children (which requires feeding them a sufficiently healthy diet) *and* having a happy, close family (which is furthered by spending quality time together on weekday evenings rather than spending that time in the kitchen). There may be significant trade-offs between meeting these ends and tensions between them, and this person may not have grappled with the trade-offs and worked out which of them are the best to make. Furthermore, from the perspective of her life plan and her conception of the good, there may be no single best way to resolve the tensions. Or perhaps there *are* better and worse ways of resolving the tensions, but this person has not discovered (yet) the better ways. People do not always respond to trade-offs in optimal ways. Sometimes they resolve dilemmas sub-optimally and act in ways that undermine their ends and their life plans.

Thus, even though unhealthy dietary patterns can represent someone making the best of the dilemmas she faces, we should not assume that unhealthy dietary patterns always represent the best response to the trade-offs and dilemmas around eating that people face in their daily lives. Unhealthy dietary patterns may be a mistake for many people; they may undermine people's life plans and conceptions of the good. And even when unhealthy dietary patterns *do* represent the best response to the contextualized trade-offs people face, there may still be a role for policy to change the social and economic context in order to reduce those trade-offs. For example, limits on junk food advertising to children might reduce their desire for junk food, which would reduce their requests to parents, which would prevent parents from having to say no to these requests. In this way, a policy can change the social context and reduce the social costs of healthier eating, thereby reducing the tension for parents between raising healthy children and having a happy, close family.

It is plausible that many people adopt unhealthy dietary patterns that really are not consistent with their life plans and conceptions of the good. Indeed, we can tell a plausible story about how dietary patterns could develop that are misaligned with people's conceptions of the good and their life plans:

- Many of us do not go through our daily lives making active choices about what to eat, based upon reflection on which eating experiences will best further our ends. What we eat often reflects habits and stable food preferences.
- The practical exigencies of life may make quicker, easier, and cheaper dietary patterns more immediately attractive. Even when these dietary patterns are less healthy and for that reason are misaligned with our long-term goals, they are the path of least resistance.
- In early childhood, long before we had a conception of the good or a life plan, we were exposed to foods and adopted certain dietary patterns. These early exposures and dietary patterns shaped our food preferences, and these preferences influence our adult dietary patterns (Hawkes et al. 2015).
- We are norm-responsive creatures, and prevalent social norms about eating—how people around us eat—influence our behaviour (Cruwys et al. 2015; Robinson et al. 2013). In very simple ways, the modes of eating we see around us affect how we eat. To give one example, larger portion sizes are linked to greater consumption (Livingstone and Pourshahidi 2014; Zlatevska et al. 2014). Plausibly we are influenced by social norms and prevalent modes of eating to adopt certain dietary patterns whether they align with our life plans or not.

- As a result of food marketing, foods high in fat, sugar, and salt are ubiquitous in our daily environments (Hawkes et al. 2015; Roberto et al. 2015; Schwartz and Brownell 2007). We have an innate liking for these foods. Eating these foods may undermine the physiological regulation of food consumption; e.g. some have argued that eating foods high in sugar and fat triggers the reward system of the brain, which reinforces the 'rewarding' behaviour (i.e. eating foods high in sugar and fat), motivating us to engage in that behaviour again and again (Kessler 2009; Roberto et al. 2015).

- Eating, as a behaviour, may not always be fully under the individual's psychological control. For example, Cohen and Farley (2008, p. 1) make the case that eating is an automatic behaviour, where automatic behaviours are those that 'occur without awareness, are initiated without intention, tend to continue without control, and operate efficiently or with little effort'. If some eating is 'initiated without intention' and is likely 'to continue without control', as Cohen and Farley suggest, we should ask whether unhealthy dietary patterns (e.g. high consumption of sugary drinks) typically reflect a choice about balancing trade-offs, or whether they are typically a kind of 'mindless eating'.

Elements of this story appear regularly in work by public health researchers and practitioners, and some are supported by empirical research (Barnhill et al. 2014; Hawkes et al. 2015; Roberto et al. 2015; Schwartz and Brownell 2007).

Thus there is evidence that dietary patterns reflect various influences and factors, including early childhood eating patterns, social norms, food marketing, and the neurophysiology of eating. We do not have reason to believe that these various influences would work to systematically align people's dietary patterns with their life plans and conceptions of the good. Thus, there is a real question about the extent to which people's unhealthy dietary patterns generally *are* aligned with their life plans and conceptions of the good. An additional piece of evidence is that most people value health, yet in some countries, many people's dietary patterns pose significant health risks; this gives us some additional reason to believe that dietary patterns can be misaligned with people's conceptions of the good.

The healthy eating efforts undertaken by public health aim to shift dietary patterns in healthier directions. Should public health assume that many people's existing patterns are *misaligned* with their life plans or their conceptions of the good, such that shifting these dietary patterns in healthier directions will, in many cases, better align dietary patterns with life plans or conceptions of the good? Or is this assumption unfounded? Should public health, on the contrary, assume that people's existing patterns are aligned with their life plans and conceptions of the good, such that shifting these dietary patterns in healthier directions may *misalign* their dietary patterns with their life plans and conceptions of the good?

Our view is that it is reasonable for public health policymakers—as a general matter—to assume that many people's unhealthy dietary patterns are misaligned with their life plans, and to assume that making dietary patterns healthier would make many people better off by their own lights. This assumption provides some ground-level justification for the public health endeavour of promoting healthy eating. But this assumption gets public health only so far. When particular healthy eating efforts are envisioned, it is important to consider how those particular efforts may affect the target population in the context of their lives. In that contextual examination, we should not simply assume that healthy eating efforts will make the target population better off all things considered. Rather, there should be consideration of the ways in which those efforts might also negatively affect individuals or upset the careful balance they are striking between eating healthfully and other ends that are central to their lives.

1.8. The upshot for this book

The analysis conducted in this chapter plays a twofold role within the context of our book. First, it shows that people's eating choices are complex and present different and often conflicting dimensions and goals. This is not only interesting from a sociological perspective and because it enriches our understanding of eating. It should also shape how we think about the normative assessment of healthy eating efforts. Focusing on a single value, such as liberty or well-being, or a single ethical concern, such as paternalism or health equity, is not sufficient when evaluating such efforts from an ethical perspective. Rather, we should be alert to potential trade-offs between these and other values, make them central to that evaluation, and use this knowledge to inform the design of such efforts. The second contribution of this chapter is therefore to indirectly introduce the theoretical and normative framework that we will develop throughout the book, and which will result in a set of policy guidelines illustrated in Chapter 7. Those guidelines will aim to help policymakers and the general public to decide whether, when, and how healthy eating efforts are publicly justified. In doing so, they will stress the importance of finding a reasonable balance between the different values at stake in the design and implementation of such efforts, and of relying on sound empirical evidence about healthy eating and the effects of healthy eating efforts.

2

Political Philosophy and Healthy Eating Efforts

Some Important Connections

2.1. Introduction

The aim of this chapter is to provide those who are not familiar with political philosophy with an understanding of how key debates in that field may have implications for the analysis of healthy eating efforts. In doing so, this chapter introduces some key terms, concepts, and theories in political philosophy that will help us to better contextualize our arguments in the following chapters.

First, we consider different conceptions of freedom in political philosophy. These include negative freedom, positive freedom, and republican freedom (or freedom as non-domination). For each of these conceptions, the chapter explores various ways in which people's eating habits, as well as governments' healthy eating efforts, may render individuals more or less free. Second, we examine the idea of democracy, especially distinguishing between aggregative (i.e. vote-centric) and deliberative conceptions. Third, we consider different conceptions of equality and justice. Fourth, we examine the relationship between theories of multiculturalism and healthy eating. And, finally, we introduce the debate on state neutrality and perfectionism, which will be a key theme throughout the remainder of the book.

2.2. Healthy eating efforts and freedom

2.2.1. Negative freedom

A first key concept from political philosophy that we would like to examine in relation to healthy eating is freedom. As we already saw in Chapter 1, when it comes to healthy eating efforts, freedom is often appealed to in order to

Healthy Eating Policy and Political Philosophy. Anne Barnhill and Matteo Bonotti, Oxford University Press. © Oxford University Press 2022. DOI: 10.1093/oso/9780190937881.003.0003

criticize any state interventions aimed at coercing people into eating more healthfully. This position is often associated with anti-paternalist arguments, i.e. arguments that challenge government efforts that aim to make the individual better off and are motivated by a negative judgement about the individual's ability to advance her own welfare and/or interfere with their freedom without their consent (Dworkin 2021; Quong 2011). We will return to the analysis of paternalism in Chapter 4. For now, we would like to stress that one way in which healthy eating efforts may be in tension with freedom is that they infringe upon what in political philosophy is called *negative* freedom, i.e. lack of interference by other agents (e.g. the state or other citizens). The idea of negative freedom has a long-standing pedigree in the history of political thought. It can already be found, e.g., in Thomas Hobbes' ([1651] 1994, Pt. 2, Chap. 21) view that 'a free man is he that in those things which by his strength and wit he is able to do is not hindered to do what he hath the will to do'. Not being hindered or interfered with is what defines this conception of freedom.

At first glance, it appears that some healthy eating efforts may restrict freedom thus intended. Food bans, that completely prevent individuals from being able to access certain foods, e.g., interfere with individuals' negative freedom. Even less coercive measures, such as sugary drink taxes, could be said to restrict individuals' negative freedom in one respect, e.g. by interfering with their freedom to buy the taxed foods if they do not have sufficient money and/or by preventing them from using some of their money to buy other things.

However, things are more complicated than appeared at first glance. Political philosophers disagree about the kind of constraints that render individuals unfree in the negative freedom sense. More specifically, some would argue that individuals are *unfree* to purchase unhealthy foods only to the extent that *other people* interfere with their freedom to do so, and that this interference is *intentional* (see Kristjánsson 1996; Miller 1983; Oppenheim 1961; Steiner 1983). These other people might be, e.g., policymakers who intentionally impose taxes on such foods. But if the key factor that prevents people from purchasing these taxed foods is the lack of sufficient financial resources, this raises a further question: Should such lack of resources be considered the result of intentional interference by others? Here political philosophers are divided. Some, especially so-called libertarians, would argue that lack of financial resources is the result of impersonal (and, therefore, unintentional) market forces, which may limit our *ability* to purchase certain goods (including more heavily taxed unhealthy foods) but not our *freedom* to do so (e.g. Hayek 1960, 1982). Others, especially so-called egalitarians, would argue instead that market forces, while apparently impersonal and unintentional, are something at least some agents are responsible for, and therefore count as restrictions on people's freedom (Cohen 1988; Crocker 1980).

Interestingly, these considerations also apply to people's negative freedom to purchase *healthy* foods (alongside taxed unhealthy foods). Indeed those who call for government subsidies for healthy foods sometimes argue that the cost of such foods may prevent lower income people from being able to purchase them. And the assumption underlying this position may be that lower income people's lack of financial resources is a condition that some other people are responsible for, and that it is therefore a form of (negative) unfreedom. Those arguing for subsidies may also assume that this kind of unfreedom (i.e. the unfreedom to buy healthy food) is unjust and that therefore governments ought to address it.

2.2.2. Positive freedom

Positive freedom is normally understood as autonomy, self-mastery, or rational self-direction, for example, as the ability to act rationally based on one's (true and authentic) desires. According to Isaiah Berlin, this conception of freedom is dangerous to the extent that its promotion may justify significant interference with our negative freedom, which, for Berlin, is the only valuable type of freedom. More specifically, Berlin (1969, pp. 132–33) argues:

> Once I take this view [i.e. that positive freedom should be promoted by advancing people's 'authentic' desires], I am in a position to ignore the actual wishes of men or societies, to bully, oppress, torture in the name, and on behalf, of their 'real' selves, in the secure knowledge that whatever is the true goal of man . . . must be identical with his freedom.

Here we will put aside the issue of whether positive freedom is dangerous. Instead, we would like to spell out the relevance of positive freedom, understood as autonomy, for the analysis of healthy eating and healthy eating efforts.

In the philosophical and practical ethics literature, there are many distinct conceptions of autonomy and claims about autonomous attitudes, choices, and actions. Some of those particularly relevant to eating and dietary patterns include the view that choice and action must be sufficiently informed in order to be autonomous; the view that preferences, choices, and actions are autonomous only if they are reflectively endorsed or would be reflectively endorsed; notions of autonomy according to which whether a preference or desire is autonomous depends upon how one came to form it, e.g. it must not be an adaptive preference formed in response to restricted options, and must not be the result of controlling influences, such as manipulation; and substantive notions of autonomy, according to which we are autonomous only if we are sufficiently responsive to reasons.

In this section, we consider how our food preferences and behaviours might fail to be free/autonomous on these views, and in particular how the influences on food preferences and behaviours discussed in the previous chapter might render us non-autonomous or unfree. When influences *do* render food preferences or behaviours unfree/non-autonomous, an important ethical question is whether the state should address these influences, with the aim of making our food preferences and behaviour freer in that sense. If so, what kinds of efforts may the state use to promote freedom in that sense?

2.2.3. Autonomous choice as requiring informed action

It is commonly claimed that for choice or action to be autonomous it must be sufficiently informed. There is a straightforward application to eating and dietary patterns: insofar as someone is not sufficiently informed about her dietary pattern and its important effects, the dietary pattern is less autonomously enacted. There is substantial evidence that people can lack basic nutritional information about the foods they consume (e.g. calorie content). Some public health experts argue that food labels do not provide clear information about the nutritional content of food, or even intentionally confuse consumers, and that as a result some consumers are poorly informed about the effects of food products on their health (Nestle and Ludwig 2010).

Thus, the key questions for healthy eating and healthy eating efforts are the following: what kinds of information deficits render dietary patterns substantially non-autonomous? What kinds of information deficits can and ought to be corrected? And with what kinds of efforts, e.g. food labelling and nutrition education?

2.2.4. Autonomy as reflective endorsement

Some views of autonomy tie it to reflective endorsement: to be autonomous and rule oneself one must have 'the capacity to reflect upon and endorse (or identify with) one's desires, values, and so on', i.e. to display 'second-order identification with first order desires' (Christman 2018). According to one version of such a view, autonomy requires actual reflective endorsement: one's desires are autonomous only if one has actually critically reflected upon them and endorsed them. For example, one's desire to have a certain dietary pattern is autonomous only if one has reflected on the likely effects of that dietary pattern (for health, family life, finances, etc.), and then reflectively endorsed one's desire to have that dietary pattern. Depending on how demanding the critical reflection must be (how informed, how well-reasoned, how comprehensive, etc.), arguably few people critically reflect on their dietary pattern as a whole and endorse it, and thus few people's dietary patterns are autonomously desired. Analogously to how a drug addict, according to this conception, is not positively free if they do not reflectively endorse the desires of their lower addicted self, someone who prefers an unhealthy dietary pattern simply because unhealthy foods are tastier and more immediately pleasant, but would not endorse this pattern if they rationally reflected upon it, is not autonomous. But so, too, someone is not autonomous who adopts a healthier dietary pattern without recognizing the (economic, social, psychological, etc.) costs of this dietary pattern, and then reflectively endorsing it despite these costs.

According to another version of the reflective endorsement view, autonomy does not require actual reflective endorsement but only *hypothetical* reflective endorsement, i.e. that one would endorse the attitude if one were to critically reflect upon it in a prescribed fashion. It is possible that many people would not reflectively endorse their unhealthy dietary patterns were they to critically reflect upon them in certain ways: if asked to critically reflect upon their unhealthy dietary patterns in light of their life plans, it is possible (even plausible?) that many people would not endorse them. For example, in the US there are relatively high rates of dieting: in the period 2013–16, half of people tried to lose weight during the previous 12 months (Martin et al. 2018). This perhaps suggests that many people have the experience of reflecting upon their dietary pattern, not endorsing it, and endeavouring to change it. It may also suggest that if other people were encouraged to engage in this reflective process, they might also fail to endorse their dietary patterns.

2.2.5. Autonomy as requiring freedom from controlling influence

On many views of autonomous choice and action, autonomy requires freedom from controlling influences—i.e. influences that render our actions non-voluntary, such as coercion (Beauchamp and Childress 2019). On these views, we are autonomous only to the extent that we engage in voluntary action and are not coerced (or exploited or manipulated) by others into having the attitudes we have, making the choices we make, and performing the actions we perform.

As discussed in the previous chapter, some work by public health researchers and advocates highlights ways in which food marketing may undermine our voluntary, deliberate control over what we eat. The food industry has engineered 'irresistible', highly palatable packaged foods, and, as a result of food marketing, these foods are ubiquitous in many people's daily environments (Moss 2013; Roberto et al. 2015; Schwartz and Brownell 2007). These highly palatable foods, we saw in the previous chapter, affect us neurophysiologically and undermine the regulation of food consumption. According to Kessler (2009), eating highly palatable foods (those high in sugar and fat) activates the reward system of the brain, which reinforces 're-warding' behaviours (food, drugs, sex, etc.), motivating us to engage in those behaviours over and over. One refrain in public health advocacy is that the food industry *exploits* our biological and neurophysiological vulnerabilities by engineering foods that are hard to resist. A related charge, illustrated in the following quote (Roberto et al. 2015, pp. 2404–5), is that food companies have intentionally engineered (or 'manipulated') foods to have this effect (see also Moss 2013):

> Incentivised to maximise profits, the food industry manipulates ingredients, such as sugar, fat, and salt, along with flavour enhancers, food additives,

and caffeine, to increase the reward value of foods. Many ultra-processed foods are also depleted of fibre and protein, two components that can enhance satiation and slow absorption of ingredients, such as sugar, into the bloodstream. Research using rats suggests that exposure to ultra-processed foods high in added sugar, fat, and salt leads to behavioural and neurobiological changes, consistent with an addictive process. Neuroimaging of human brains has also shown that food intake and drug use trigger similar brain activity. This biological vulnerability to ultra-processed foods is especially concerning for children because they have a stronger preference for sweet foods than do adults.

Along with manipulating the ingredients of foods, the food industry is charged with engaging in manipulative advertising practices (Paynter 2019). Commercial advertising, more generally, is often claimed to be manipulative (Sunstein 2016; Wood 2014). Though it is often unclear what kinds of complaints are being registered by a particular charge of manipulation, charges of manipulation generally register one of four distinct kinds of concerns and complaints: first, that the (purportedly) manipulative influence bypasses the influenced person's rationality, fails to sufficiently engage their rationality, or undermines their practical reasoning (for example, Farley 2015 refers to food marketing that 'bypasses our rational minds'); second, that the influence undermines its target's self-control in a problematic way; third, that the influence is covert or sneaky; and fourth, that the influence targets the influenced person's weaknesses or vulnerabilities (see Barnhill 2014; Coons and Weber 2014). On this understanding of manipulation, much food advertising is, arguably, manipulative: it intentionally fails to engage us in reflection about food choices and instead plays on our emotions and impulses and leverages social norms; it contributes to failures of self-control vis-à-vis eating; it influences us in ways that we do not understand or recognize; and it targets our psychological vulnerabilities (Barnhill 2016; Sunstein 2016). Whether manipulation of these sorts undermines voluntary choice—and thus undermines autonomous choice—is a separate and complicated question; it hinges on how we understand voluntary choice. Interestingly, the issue of manipulation is also relevant to the promotion of *healthy* eating. For example, just as commercial marketing of food may be manipulative, so, too, public health messaging that promotes healthy eating—which deploys some of the same techniques as commercial marketing—may also be manipulative, an argument that some public health ethicists have advanced (Faden 1987).

Wikler (1978, p. 329), e.g., raises the concern that '[s]uggestion and manipulation may replace information as the tools used by the health educators to accomplish their purpose . . . These measures bypass rational decision-making faculties and thereby inflict a loss of personal control'. Guttman and Salmon (2004, p. 532) note that '[f]or centuries, governments and other social institutions have engaged communication strategies in the service of public health through tactics some may consider to be "benevolent public manipulation"'. The philosopher Allen Wood (2014, p. 38) takes aim at all advertising, including commercial advertising and public health messaging:

> Advertisements use constant repetition to wear down our resistance, to reinforce associations at a subrational level, to offer us inducements that are illusory or otherwise 'of the wrong sort' . . . Even advertisements that manipulate people for what we might think are good ends—to vote for the right candidates, to give up smoking—do it in bad ways. Advertising never aims to convince, only to persuade. It corrupts the root of rational communication, precludes the possibility of any free human community.

The charge of manipulation has also been raised against healthy eating efforts that make use of nudges, i.e. efforts to change behaviour without limiting or penalizing options, such as putting healthy foods first in a cafeteria line (Thaler and Sunstein 2008). Nudges are considered manipulative by some theorists, and some ethical objections to nudges repeat the main ethical complaints with manipulation: nudges are seen as a potentially problematic form of control or as exploiting people's rational failings or failing to treat them as rational agents (Conly 2013a; Eyal 2016; Hausman and Welch 2010; Waldron 2014). For example, critics argue that by '[s]ystematically exploiting non-rational factors that influence human decision-making, whether on the part of the government or other agents, [nudges threaten] liberty, broadly conceived' (Hausman and Welch 2010, p. 136). In more recent work, Noggle (2018) considers nudges that modify the salience of different options available to people. He distinguishes between salience nudges that exert pressure on people's choices ('pressure' nudges) and those that trick people into making certain choices ('trickery' nudges), concluding that only the latter are manipulative. In response to these concerns, some have argued that various forms of counter-manipulation could be employed to prevent or counteract wrongful manipulative public health efforts, thus protecting or restoring people's autonomy (Wilkinson 2017). However, even if nudges are manipulative in some sense, or fail to fully engage our rationality in some sense, it is a separate question whether they render our actions and choices non-voluntary and thus non-autonomous.

2.2.6. Adaptive preferences

Adaptive preferences are preferences formed in conditions of deprivation or restriction of options, and which may seem to reflect that deprivation. An example from the literature is the preferences of women who live in patriarchal societies that deny basic opportunities to them; a woman might come to prefer not to have equal political rights or education, own property, or be employed outside the home, and even to prefer that lot for her daughters (Khader 2011; Nussbaum 2001). The woman might reflectively endorse these preferences and the choices she makes based on them; nonetheless, these preferences and choices may not seem fully free and autonomous. In addition, fulfilment of these preferences may not seem, intuitively, to promote or constitute women's welfare. Another, somewhat different category of adaptive preferences—sometimes called 'sour grapes' preferences—consists of preferences that change in response to people's options being restricted (Elster 1983), as in 'I didn't want that stupid job anyway' or 'I now see how terrible my ex is, and I'm better off without them'. People may adapt their preferences to their current situation because they realize that other alternatives are precluded. These preferences, too, might not seem fully free and autonomous, even if they are reflectively endorsed, and fulfilment of these preferences may seem not to promote someone's welfare.

Might some food preferences be adaptive preferences? Consider a consumer who does not have enough money to afford a diet of healthier foods, and in these conditions develops preferences for the less healthy foods and dietary pattern that she can afford. Arguably these are preferences formed under restricted options, and thus should not be considered fully free and autonomous preferences in some sense. In addition to financial resources limiting food options, commercial food marketing could also be said to limit our options, in a sense, since food marketing may function to occlude other options. Some work critical of food industry influence argues that the food industry presents consumers with a set of low-quality options— e.g. processed foods high in sugar, salt, and fat—aggressively markets these options, and has pervaded everyday environments with these foods and food marketing (see e.g. Schwartz and Brownell 2007). If consumers develop preferences for these foods, and for dietary patterns high in these foods, should these be seen as adaptive preferences formed in conditions of limited or restricted options? And if food preferences are adaptive preferences caused by food marketing, what does this imply for the government's warrant to regulate food marketing?

In claiming that food preferences are adaptive preferences, however, we need to be careful. Some critical work on healthy eating efforts argues that these efforts, insofar as they assume that people's food behaviour is the result of environmental influences, are undergirded by a belittling or scornful attitude towards people. For example, Julie Guthman (2007, p. 78) writes:

> That, then, is the most pernicious aspect of the [Michael] Pollan et al. analysis. If junk food is everywhere and people are all naturally drawn to it, those who resist it must have heightened powers. In the reality television show *The Biggest Loser,* where fat people compete to lose the most weight (about which much could be said), the contestants are treated paternalistically; the hard-body trainers are treated as super-subjects who readily and regularly bestow life wisdom on their charges. So when Pollan waxes poetic about his own rarefied, distinctive eating practices, he makes a similar move. The messianic quality and self-satisfaction is not accidental. In describing his ability to overcome King Corn, to conceive, procure, prepare, and (perhaps) serve his version of the perfect meal, Pollan affirms himself as a super-subject while relegating others to objects of education, intervention, or just plain scorn.

In a similar vein, Anna Kirkland (2011) discerns in healthy eating efforts a belittling attitude towards low-income people. Efforts focused on increasing access to healthy foods assume that low-income people would prefer to eat more healthfully, if only they had better access to healthy food; these efforts do not take seriously the fact that people's eating practises might reflect their actual preferences.

Though these authors do not use the language of 'adaptive preferences', plausibly they would approach the claim that people's food preferences are adaptive preferences with the same scepticism as the claim that people's food behaviour is environmentally determined: who are we to assume that people's preferences are adaptive, rather than preferences that reflect the person's life plans or conception of the good? Therefore, generally speaking, we need to ensure that we do not make unwarranted assumptions about people's preferences, such as assuming that these are adaptive preferences formed in response to deprivation rather than preferences reflecting the person's ends and conception of the good. A way to safeguard against these assumptions would be to put mechanisms in place to understand what people's preferences are, how they came to have those preferences, and how they understand those preferences. Such mechanisms could include social science research or the kind of deliberative forums discussed later in this book.

Another perspective on the food industry and on how it has influenced us is also relevant here. Plausibly, the food industry has changed our preferences, our expectations, our norms, and perhaps even our underlying values about food (Barnhill 2016). The food industry has produced a range of products—packaged foods, convenience foods, heat-and-eat meals, sugary foods, snack foods—and introduced food marketing strategies that have, over time, altered our gustatory preferences (e.g. we now favour sweeter and saltier food), influenced our expectations regarding food and food preparation (e.g. we are less inclined to spend much time preparing food, and we demand cheaper food), and shaped our social norms regarding food (e.g. we now consider larger serving sizes as normal) (Bittman 2013, 2014; Freedhoff 2015; Pollan 2006). Commetators argue that these changes to our preferences, expectations, and norms are not positive. They are good for food companies but bad for us: they have steered us towards preferences for products and eating styles that render us unhealthy, displacing healthier and more meaningful eating styles, such as those that involve preparing and eating home-cooked meals (Bittman 2014; Freedhoff 2015; Kingsolver et al. 2008). For example, we have come to expect and value convenience, even though spending time on making and eating food is actually a highly valuable experience (Kingsolver et al. 2008). Therefore, some commentators seem to be arguing that the way in which the food industry influences us is not just by undermining our ability to make choices based on our food preferences (i.e. by undermining our voluntary control over our eating or by manipulating our behaviour, as discussed in the previous section), but also by changing what we prefer, what we expect, and what we find normative.

2.2.7. Substantive conceptions of autonomy

On another conception of autonomy, our preferences (including our food preferences) are non-autonomous if they are insufficiently responsive to reasons (e.g. see Berofsky 1995; Meyers 1989). On this view, autonomy is not just a matter of endorsing one's attitudes, choices, or actions, or forming them through a certain kind of process (i.e. a process that is free of controlling influence by others); autonomy requires that the agent recognizes and responds to the reasons that actually bear on her attitudes, choices, or actions. On this view, unhealthy dietary patterns could be assessed as non-autonomous if they are not sufficiently responsive to the relevant reasons, which would include reasons to adopt a healthy dietary pattern as well as reasons not to. It is worth noting that on some versions of this view, the reasons that the autonomous agent must be responsive to are subjective reasons (reasons the agent has in light of her preferences, ends, and conception of the good), and on other versions they are objective reasons.

2.2.8. Republican freedom

Another major conception of freedom is the republican idea of freedom as non-domination. Unlike 'negative' freedom, which signals the absence of actual (or imminent) interference by others, and 'positive' freedom, which involves autonomy and self-mastery, non-domination refers to the absence of 'arbitrary' (Pettit 1997) or 'uncontrolled' (Pettit 2012) interference or mastery by others. According to Pettit, a person enjoys non-domination if she is not subject to institutional, legal, and social factors that render the exercise of her rights and negative liberties insecure and dependent on other agents' unpredictable interference (even if such interference never becomes actual). Pettit's idea of 'uncontrolled' interference shifts the focus from arbitrariness to 'interference that is exercised at the will or discretion of the interferer; interference that is uncontrolled by the person on the receiving end' (Pettit 2012, p. 58). This shift of focus is necessary, according to Pettit, because even when there are non-arbitrary rules in place, 'interference that conforms to rules, and is not arbitrary in that sense, may still be uncontrolled by you and can count as arbitrary in our sense' (p. 58). Individuals who are non-dominated enjoy 'security in the exercise of ... [their] basic liberties' (Pettit 2014, p. 77) and, therefore, 'the status or dignity of the free republican citizen' (p. 61).

The aforementioned criticism against nudges can be reformulated on the basis of this conception: nudges, including healthy eating nudges, not only prevent us from engaging in rational self-rule (the idea central to a positive conception of freedom), in virtue of failing to engage our rationality, but may also involve alien, arbitrary, and uncontrolled influence by policymakers. Yet this is only one half of the story. State-sponsored healthy eating nudges are normally not implemented against a background of non-dominating influences on consumers. The food industry uses many different kinds of (dominating) nudges in order to influence consumers' food choices; an example is situating products in prominent locations in grocery stores to encourage consumers to purchase them. And even the shape of glasses in which drinks (including alcoholic drinks) are served can increase the amount of drink we consume. A study showed, e.g., that people consume an alcoholic drink from a straight glass more slowly than from a curved glass (Attwood et al. 2012). State-sponsored healthy eating nudges, including greater use of straight-sided glasses (Langfield et al. 2020), could therefore be reconceived as 'counter-nudges', whose moral permissibility is strengthened if they are transparent and democratically controlled by citizens (see Schmidt 2017).

The republican idea of freedom as non-domination also helps us to capture another issue related to healthy eating efforts. Central to republican freedom is not only the idea of non-domination but also the importance of choice. According to Pettit (2014, p. 29), '[y]ou must be able to get what you want regardless of what others want you to get. Your freedom in this sense must have depth'. Arguably some people lack sufficient choice of healthy eating options, e.g. people who do not have access to stores that sell a range of healthy foods. This lack of choice depends on structural factors, such as technological and infrastructural ones, e.g. lack of grocery stores in their neighbourhood and/or lack of affordable private or public transport enabling them to travel to such outlets if these are distant from their home. Increasing food choice for people living in these areas will require addressing these structural problems, e.g. through the redistribution of material resources, state support for infrastructure and public transport, etc. Furthermore, since the food industry is increasingly controlled by multinational food corporations, non-domination requires the establishment and/or strengthening of international agencies regulating food production, distribution, and consumption that are subject to citizens' democratic control and contestation and that follow impartial rules (Bonotti 2020a).

2.3. Healthy eating efforts and democracy

In the previous section we anticipated a theme that deserves separate attention: the relationship between healthy eating efforts and democracy.

Democracy, understood as collective self-government or self-rule, is often considered a type of positive freedom. In the same way in which individuals are positively free (i.e. autonomous) when they are self-ruling, a collective body of citizens is democratic when each of its members has had the opportunity to contribute to shaping the laws and policies all of them are subject to. Focusing on democracy in relation to healthy eating efforts is important since debates on such policies tend to focus on individuals qua consumers whose negative or positive freedom is at stake (as we saw in the previous section) rather than as citizens involved in processes of collectively binding decision-making (Ankeny 2016). What is then, more exactly, the relevance of democracy to debates on healthy eating efforts?

First, it is important to stress that democracy comes in many forms. An important distinction is that between aggregative and deliberative models of democracy. The former is centred around voting and involves the aggregation of individuals' preferences, mediated by various kinds of decision-making procedures (electoral systems, majority rule, etc.) in order to produce collective decisions. The latter requires going beyond mere voting to include processes of deliberation through which citizens debate key policies and, by exchanging reasons and drawing on available evidence, reach a consensus on key policy decisions or recommendations. Defenders of deliberative democracy argue that the latter ensures procedural fairness (Benhabib 1996; Cohen 1996), produces better policies (Habermas 1996), educates citizens to skills like other-regardingness and respect for other people's views (Gutmann and Thompson 1996), and helps them to better understand, articulate, and justify their own preferences and values (Chambers 1996; Niemeyer 2011). All of this can contribute to more legitimate and effective policy (for a survey of these debates, see Bächtiger et al. 2018; Bohman 1998; Chappell 2012; Gastil and Levine 2005).

Aggregative democracy can certainly play an important role with regard to healthy eating efforts, by ensuring that consumers, qua citizens, play an active role in shaping such efforts (sugary drink taxes, nudges, laws regulating food marketing, etc.). One problem with this model of democracy, however, is that it tends to take people's preferences as given. When people vote in referendums or elections, that is, many of them normally vote based on their given or unreflective preferences with regard to different policies, even if such preferences are misguided, misinformed, or resulting from various forms of manipulation. For example, if the food industry, through its marketing strategies, persuades me that eating fast foods every day is not unhealthy, then in a referendum about a proposed tax on fast foods I may vote against this measure for that reason.

Deliberative democracy aims to answer this kind of challenge. When citizens are asked to engage in deliberative forums, they may be presented with evidence concerning, say, the nutritional content of fast foods, the effect of such foods on human health in the short and long term, the various ways in which the food industry is able to shape people's preferences through marketing, nudging, etc. At the same time, however, citizens in such forums may also be asked to deliberate on the ethical issues at stake when it comes to a proposed fast-food tax. For example, even once all deliberating parties have been informed about the potential effects of fast foods on health, and even if they agree that fast foods are unhealthy, disagreements concerning the permissibility of a fast-food tax may still remain. A person, e.g., may accept that evidence while still believing that other values (e.g. short-term pleasure or conviviality) are more important for them than long-term health, and that therefore a fast-food tax is not justifiable all things considered. Different participants in deliberation may hold different views on these ethical issues, and they could sometimes be helped by professional ethicists to carry out an informed discussion about them. Since deliberation is normally aimed at achieving some kind of consensus, it is important that participants reach decisions or recommendations about a policy that are grounded in reasons all of them would be able to accept at some general level. However, when that is not possible, resorting to aggregative forms of decision-making (i.e. voting) may be the only option left.

Somewhere between aggregative and deliberative forms of democracy we can find the republican conception of democracy. Republicans do not normally endorse demanding participatory or deliberative forms of democracy. For them, democracy primarily requires control and contestation over political decisions (Pettit 2012). This involves, of course, elections but also contestatory tools such as public interest bodies which give voice to consumers vis-à-vis producers, including food producers and multinational food corporations (Bonotti 2020a).

The idea of democracy, in its various understandings, also captures an important aspect of 'food sovereignty', i.e. 'the right of people to *healthy* and culturally appropriate food produced through ecologically sound and sustainable methods, and their right to define their own food and agriculture systems' (La Via Campesina 2007, emphasis added). According to advocates of food sovereignty, this requires that communities have a right to self-government: '[t]o demand a space of food sovereignty is to demand specific arrangements to govern territory and space' (Patel 2009, p. 668). The connection between healthy eating and democratic self-government is an important one under food sovereignty. It implies that healthy eating efforts cannot be decided on behalf of specific communities, but that the latter should have the right to deliberate and decide about them, in ways which, as we will explain later, are also consistent with their cultural habits.

2.4. Healthy eating efforts, equality, and justice

We already pointed out, in our discussion of freedom, that there are a variety of financial, social, environmental, and personal factors that affect our freedom to eat healthfully. These can be examined, e.g., through the lens of effective negative freedom or freedom as non-domination. But issues concerning these factors can also be analysed in connection with another key idea in political philosophy, that of equality. We need to ask, i.e. not only what it means for an individual to be free to eat healthfully but also what it means for eating, and healthy eating, to conform to principles of equality. Like freedom, equality is also a complex concept which can be understood in very different ways. Here we consider different views about equality and muse about what might be required for these principles to be fulfiled vis-à-vis healthy eating.

2.4.1. Equality of opportunity

One principle or ideal of equality is equality of opportunity. According to a basic conception, equality of opportunity means 'careers open to talents', in other words, 'positions and posts that confer superior advantages should be open to all applicants. Applications are assessed on their merits, and the applicant deemed most qualified according to appropriate criteria is offered the position' (Arneson 2015).

While apparently straightforward, this conception raises a number of complex questions (Arneson 2015). A key issue that has significant implications for healthy eating policy concerns what is perhaps the most fundamental limit of formal equality of opportunity. This is the fact that, even if careers and other desirable positions are allocated based on merit, some people may be more able than others to become meritorious. If a society is characterized by some kind of social hierarchy, and merit is more easily obtained by people in certain positions in this social hierarchy, then some people will be more meritorious than others, i.e. more able than others to access careers and opportunities that are formally open to all. This might happen, e.g., if '[e]veryone in society except the wealthy is poorly nourished, and being well nourished is a prerequisite' (Arneson 2015) for succeeding in competitive selection processes, e.g. to join the military or acquire other types of key positions.

This situation strikes some theorists as a failure of equality of opportunity and motivates what is labelled 'substantive equality of opportunity', according to which 'all [should] have a genuine opportunity to become qualified' (Arneson 2015). This genuine opportunity would include opportunities to be educated, of course, and the opportunity to eat healthfully or to access '[n]utrition supplements [that] are made available to those whose diet is inadequate' (Arneson 2015), given the importance of good nutrition and health to mental and physical functioning in general, and to learning in particular.

Therefore, there seem to be two dimensions of equality of opportunity clearly related to healthy eating. On the one hand, there is what we could call opportunities *for* healthy eating, i.e. opportunities to eat healthfully, which may be affected by such diverse factors as one's financial resources or one's family. On the other hand, we find opportunities *from* healthy eating, i.e. opportunities that we can access when we have access to healthy eating, e.g. opportunities for physical health, better performance in school, better jobs, or success in sports competitions. These constitute the two sides of equality of opportunity when it comes to healthy eating.

But what does it mean, exactly, to have 'a genuine opportunity to become qualified', e.g. in our case to have a genuine opportunity to eat healthfully and, as a result, be able to access other opportunities? The most influential response to this question is that provided by John Rawls through the idea of *fair* equality of opportunity. According to Rawls (1999, p. 63), fair equality of opportunity can be understood in the following way: 'assuming there is a distribution of natural assets, those who are at the same level of talent and ability, and have the same willingness to use them . . . have the same prospects of success regardless of their initial place in the social system'.

Building on this, Norman Daniels has offered what is probably the most influential analysis of the relationship between health and fair equality of opportunity. Daniels draws on Rawls' view in order to justify the provision of healthcare for individuals. According to him, 'impairments of normal functioning reduce the range of exercisable opportunities from which individuals may construct their "plans of life" or "conceptions of the good"' (Daniels 2008, p. 35). If two individuals have the same talents and skills, but any social factors (wealth, race, etc.) have unequally affected their ability to be healthy, the state should intervene and rectify that inequality, e.g. through the provision of universal healthcare. For the same reasons, one might argue, a state needs to implement healthy eating efforts in order to redress inequalities of opportunity to eat healthfully.

The problem with fair equality of opportunity, in general and when applied to healthy eating policy more specifically, is that it not only demands the aforementioned measures to provide lower-income people with affordable healthy foods; it might also demand something more. Fair equality of opportunity, recall, requires that people with the same inborn talents and motivation have 'the same prospects of success, regardless of their initial place in the social system' (Rawls 1999, p. 63). Securing this, some have observed, may require extensive interventions within family life, in order to prevent parents from raising their children in ways that impart advantages to them and help them stand out when they compete for various kinds of jobs and other opportunities (Fishkin 1983). For example, parents might provide their children with an unusually excellent education, which better develops their inborn talents and puts them in a better position to compete for jobs and other opportunities, even as compared to children with the same level of motivation and inborn talent. When it comes to healthy eating, it is clear that parents' resources and decisions significantly affect their children's diet, and therefore their children's nutrition and health, and thereby affect further opportunities that healthy eating and good nutrition would help the children to access. If some children have poor nutrition, impaired mental and physical functioning, and less ability to learn and perform well at school, they will not be able to develop their inborn talents as well as children with adequate nutrition, amounting to a failure of fair equality of opportunity. So, too, if some children have unusually good nutrition and perform usually well at school, and are better able to develop their inborn talents, this is a failure of fair equality of opportunity.

Here it seems that we face two problems. First, we need to decide whether interventions aimed at guaranteeing fair equality of opportunity should focus on levelling up or down. The former option seems prima facie better; i.e. we should not prevent, say, wealthier parents from investing in their children's education and providing them with advantages but rather help lower income parents to offset those advantages, e.g. via state-funded education and other types of interventions:

> In principle, society could allow parents to act pretty much as they please and simultaneously maintain in place flexible policies that adjust the social provision of aid to children so that whatever parents do that would result in nonfulfillment of FEO [fair equality of opportunity] if its impact were left standing is entirely offset, so the end result is that FEO is completely fulfilled. If wealthy parents give their children special tennis lessons and fancy tutorial assistance, social agencies increase aid to children whose parents do not or cannot lavish such resources on their upbringing, so the inequality-boosting tendency of the special parental provision is entirely nullified. In principle no limits on parental freedom would be needed to achieve FEO completely (though limits on secret parental helps might need to be curbed, and what might strike us as privacy-violating intrusions on family life to monitor effects of special parental provision would be needed). This possible public policy stance sounds bizarre only because its costs would clearly be enormous, and arguably not worth the moral gain in extra fulfillment of FEO they would achieve. (Arneson 2015)

When it comes to healthy eating, one might argue in this vein that the state should provide lower income children with access to free healthy foods during the school day (such as free breakfast and lunch), and through schools provide children with adequate food for the weekends and holidays, or provide their parents with food vouchers that can be used to purchase only healthy foods, e.g. fruit and vegetables. Admittedly the cost of these kinds of 'levelling up' policies, as pointed out by Arneson, could be significant.[1]

---

[1] Full levelling up might be really prohibitively expensive, at least in the US. There is a wealth-longevity gradient in the US that never levels off: the richer you are, the longer you live, and there is no level of wealth after which longevity is stationary (Chetty et al. 2016).

In addition, the financial cost of healthier foods is only one kind of cost of healthier eating, as discussed in Chapter 1. Healthier eating can also require more time and more control over one's work schedule (so that one can cook meals) and can have interpersonal and social costs. While the time and effort costs of healthy eating are in principle modifiable by public policy (e.g. the state could subsidize ready-to-eat healthy meals), it is not clear how public policy could fully address the social or interpersonal costs.

In addition, both 'levelling up' and 'levelling down' approaches could involve levels of interference with the family and with personal behaviour that many would consider morally unjustifiable. For example, in the case of 'levelling up' approaches to childhood nutrition, parents would be required to use resources in specific ways (i.e. to use food vouchers only to buy healthy foods for children). In the case of 'levelling down' interventions, parents would be stopped from feeding their children an unusually nutritious diet. Many would find either intervention, or both, highly problematic.

Does this mean that we should abandon fair equality of opportunity? Some theorists have suggested that we should abandon fair equality of opportunity in favour of an alternative, e.g. formal equality of opportunity ('careers open to talents') accompanied by 'good enough opportunities for all its members to develop their native talents so as to become qualified for competitive positions' (Arneson 2015), a position that combines a sufficientarian element ('good enough') with the formal egalitarian one. This might demand providing people with a good enough opportunity to access healthy eating, without aiming to redress all inequalities in this area. But what does a 'good enough opportunity to eat healthfully' imply? What does it consist of, and require? Any answer to this question is likely to be contested.

2.4.2. Pluralizing opportunities

There is another alternative to fair equality of opportunity, advanced by Fishkin (2014). Rather than embarking on the admittedly demanding task of redressing any inequalities that affect fair equality of opportunity, one might focus on pluralizing opportunities. The problem in liberal democracies, according to this view, is often that institutional requirements and/or social norms demand that one meets certain criteria or passes through certain 'bottlenecks' (Fishkin 2014) in order to access certain opportunities. By pluralizing the routes to opportunities, e.g. by not requiring all children to pass a single test at a certain age in order to be able to access job and educational prospects, a society may broaden people's access to opportunities.

When it comes to healthy eating this may imply, amongst other things, moving beyond a narrow understanding of health and well-being, which focuses purely on physical health, and understanding that health and well-being, for children and adults alike, involve other aspects that may sometimes be in conflict with physical health, understood as the absence of disease. While this does not mean that the latter should be dismissed, the question arises whether physical health should always be prioritized over any other values. In other words, if some (wealthier) families focus mainly on promoting their children's physical health through healthy eating, this may of course require, to some extent, helping other (poorer) families to also secure their children's physical health in this way. However, it may also require sending the message to all citizens that physical health should not always be their priority, and that engaging (and encouraging one's children to engage) in some consumption of unhealthy foods, e.g. if this promotes their well-being by fostering cultural, social, and religious values, is often acceptable and should not be penalized (e.g. through weight stigma and other negative social norms that may affect children's opportunities). This requires an overall rethinking of the relationship between healthy eating and equality of opportunity (for a more detailed analysis of these issues, see Bonotti and Calder 2021).

2.4.3. Healthy eating and sufficientarianism

In contrast to theories arguing that justice requires an equal distribution of some sort (e.g. an equal distribution of opportunities), there are theories arguing that justice requires sufficiency—attainment of a sufficient level of something. For example, according to Madison Powers and Ruth Faden (2006), the positive aim of social justice should be to ensure that everyone has a *sufficient* level of well-being, where health is one dimension of well-being.

However, it is not really possible to ensure that people have a sufficient level of health, since health is affected by many factors outside of our control (genetics, chance, etc.). Therefore, the aim of justice cannot be exactly to ensure a sufficient level of health, but instead something else—e.g. to ensure a sufficient opportunity to attain an adequate level of health. What might this imply for healthy eating? There is a strong connection between diet and health; thus, one might argue that ensuring sufficient opportunity to be healthy requires ensuring sufficient opportunity to *eat* healthfully. It would then be a complicated matter, once again, to spell out what amounts to a sufficient opportunity to eat healthfully.

2.4.4. Health equity and structural injustice

We have just considered three conceptions of justice. Actual societies may fail, and typically do fail, to conform to these conceptions of justice.[2] One way in which societies so fail is that they are marked by deep and pervasive social disadvantages—i.e. unfavourable social, economic, or political conditions that some groups systematically experience as a result of group membership (Braveman et al. 2011). In the high-income liberal democracies that are our focus in this book, systematically disadvantaged groups include people of colour, indigenous people and ethnic minorities, people of some genders (e.g. transgender people, women and girls in general, gender-nonconforming people), religious minorities, lower-income people, and people with disabilities, to give just some examples.

Systematic disadvantage can take the form of structural injustice, i.e. injustice in which some groups occupy disfavourable positions within a self-reinforcing social structure.[3] One manifestation of structural injustice is significant differences across groups in the *social determinants of health*—i.e. 'the conditions in which people are born, grow, work, live, and age, and the wider set of forces and systems shaping the conditions of daily life' (WHO 2020). Social determinants of health are various and include environmental conditions (e.g. the presence or absence of pollution), the features of neighbourhoods (e.g. whether neighbourhoods are safe or walkable, whether there is a high density of fast-food restaurants), and access to key resources (e.g. healthcare, healthy food).

---

[2] Indeed, on any conception of justice, including non-egalitarian conceptions of justice, actual societies typically do fail to conform to the relevant principles of justice.

[3] We understand structural injustice in this way: there is a social system in which a variety of social phenomena (social attitudes and norms, social practices, laws and public policies, institutional practices, a material distribution of resources, and other social phenomena) are connected and work together in self-reinforcing ways, sometimes locking each other in place; different groups occupy different positions within this social structure; and some groups' positions in this social structure are disadvantaged relative to other groups' positions, in a way that is unfair and unjust. Political philosophy in the Western tradition has generally given short shrift to structural injustice, with some notable exceptions (Mills 2018; Powers and Faden 2006, 2019; Young 1990), though the tide may be turning.

For example, Bailey et al. (2017) consider the relationships between structural racism and health inequalities across racial groups in the US, and identify multiple pathways between structural racism and health inequalities. In other words, they identify both broad and specific manifestations of structural racism that causally contribute to health inequalities. These pathways between structural racism and health inequalities include forms of economic injustice and social deprivation (such as 'residential, educational, and occupational segregation of marginalised, racialised groups to low-quality neighbourhoods, schools, and jobs' (Bailey et al. 2017, p. 1456)), psychosocial trauma (e.g. from interpersonal racial discrimination and from being exposed to racist media coverage), and targeted marketing of substances that are harmful to one's health (e.g. cigarettes or sugar-sweetened beverages). In other words, structural racism profoundly affects the conditions in which people live and work, and this translates into inequalities in health behaviour and health outcomes across racial/ethnic groups.

The same could be said of economic injustice more generally, whether or not it is linked to structural racism. A large body of evidence shows significant relationships between both income and educational attainment and health behaviours and health outcomes (Braveman et al. 2010; Braveman and Gottlieb 2014). There are likely many pathways whereby income and education (via other social determinants of health) affect health behaviours and health outcomes. Some of these pathways are direct and short-term (e.g. 'lead ingestion in substandard housing contributes to low cognitive function and stunted physical development in exposed children'), whereas others are more indirect and long-term (e.g. there is a correlation between duration of childhood poverty and cognitive function in adulthood, which in turn may affect health behaviour) (Braveman and Gottlieb 2014, pp. 22–23).

Turning to food in particular, there are documented group-based differences in social determinants of health connected to eating and food. For example, in the US in 2018, 4.1% of households experienced very low food security (US Department of Agriculture [USDA] 2020). However, very low food insecurity was experienced by 4.9% of Hispanic households, 7.6% of Black, non-Hispanic households, and 9.6% of households headed by a single woman (USDA 2020).[4] To give another example, in the US, racial and ethnic minorities and socio-economically disadvantaged people have higher exposure to advertising of unhealthy foods (Backholer et al. 2020; Grier and

[4] Very low food security is defined as 'normal eating patterns of one or more household[s] [where] members were disrupted and food intake was reduced at times during the year because they had insufficient money or other resources for food' (USDA 2020).

Kumanyika 2010). In some cases, inequalities in the social determinants of healthy eating can be traced back to specific historical injustices; e.g. past housing discrimination in the US (a form of institutional racism) has resulted in African-Americans disproportionately living in areas with less access to healthy food (Braveman et al. 2011; Kumanyika 2005).

These differences in the social determinants of health—insofar as they are rooted in forms of injustice—are themselves a justice issue. That is, if you have less access to food partly as a result of your society's housing authorities enacting racist policies in the past, your worse access to food is an injustice in and of itself. But inequalities in the social determinants of health have additional importance insofar as they contribute to health inequalities between groups. That is, your worse access to food has additional importance if it contributes to your having worse health than people who are not negatively impacted by past racist policies. We do, in fact, see inequalities in diet-related illness across racial/ethnic groups and socio-economic groups. For example, in the US, there are higher rates of diabetes amongst people with less educational attainment as compared to those with greater educational attainment, and amongst Black (11.7%), Hispanic (12.5%), and Asian (9.2%) as compared to white (7.5%) people (Centers for Disease Control and Prevention [CDC] 2020a, p. 4). Also in the US, there are higher rates of overweight and obesity amongst some minority racial/ethnic groups, and lower rates of obesity amongst adults with college degrees as compared to those without (CDC 2020b).

Insofar as these health inequalities between groups are a result, at least in part, of background injustice, addressing these inequalities is a way to partially address that injustice. Thus, there are justice-based reasons to enact efforts that address the forms of background injustice that cause health inequalities (e.g. structural racism, economic injustice) and to address the specific manifestations of background injustice that may affect health (i.e. worse food access amongst many communities of colour).

In addition, even if health inequalities between groups are not the *result* of background injustice, or cannot be established as such, they still matter from the perspective of justice (Braveman et al. 2011). Health inequalities can function to lock in disadvantage and stymie efforts to address it. For example, poor nutrition and poor health may undermine children's performance in school, and this may worsen their future job prospects and future earnings. As Braveman et al. (2011, p. S150) put it, '[h]ealth differences adversely affecting socially disadvantaged groups are particularly unacceptable because ill health can be an obstacle to overcoming social disadvantage'. Thus some argue that there is a justice-based case to address health inequalities when these inequalities affect socially disadvantaged groups, whether or not we are able to establish that these inequalities are caused by background injustice (Braveman et al. 2011).

Broadly speaking, there is significant attention in public health research and practice on identifying and addressing health inequities (i.e. health inequalities between groups that are unjust), including health disparities (i.e. health inequalities that are to the disadvantage of socially disadvantaged groups). In the US, there is increasing interest in understanding how structural racism affects health and creates health inequalities, including inequalities in overweight and obesity rates (Aaron and Stanford 2021; Bailey et al. 2017; Bleich and Ard 2021). This brief discussion has attempted to provide a vindicating explanation of that focus, by explaining how there are multiple kinds of justice-based reasons to address such health inequalities.[5]

2.5. Healthy eating efforts and multiculturalism

A further area of political philosophy that is relevant to the analysis of healthy eating efforts concerns multiculturalism. Rooted in such diverse phenomena as postcolonialism, the revival of ethnocultural nationalism (in Quebec, Scotland, Catalonia, etc.), and increasing migration and globalization, multiculturalism is the idea that the cultural diversity that characterizes liberal democracies should be embraced and promoted. Multiculturalists therefore reject assimilationist policies and tend to focus especially on the importance of minority group rights (e.g. the rights of indigenous peoples, sub-state national minorities, and immigrant groups) rather than universal individual rights. Different rationales for multiculturalism have been provided in the literature. Perhaps the two most influential ones are those provided by Charles Taylor and Will Kymlicka.

Taylor defends a *communitarian* type of multiculturalism. According to this view, it is important that a state recognizes different cultures because

> our identity is partly shaped by recognition or its absence, often by the misrecognition of others, and so a person or group of people can suffer real

---

[5] For a detailed theory of social justice and structural justice in which addressing systematic disadvantage and its health impacts has a central place, see Powers and Faden (2006, 2019).

damage, real distortion, if the people or society around them mirror back to them a confining or demeaning contemptible picture of themselves. (Taylor [1992] 1994, p. 25)

If, for example, someone is a French-speaking Quebecois or an Aboriginal Australian, but their state and fellow citizens consider them simply a Canadian or an Australian, setting aside their particular cultural identities (or, worse, misrecognizing them as an Anglo-Canadian or an Anglo-European Australian), this amounts to a form of harmful non-recognition or misrecognition.

According to Kymlicka's (1989, 1995) liberal strand of multiculturalism, cultures are important not because of the intrinsic communitarian value highlighted by Taylor but because cultures and cultural contexts are instrumental to individuals' exercise of autonomy: '[i]t's only through having a rich and secure cultural structure', Kymlicka (1989, p. 165) argues, 'that people can become aware, in a vivid way, of the options available to them, and intelligently examine their value'.

Both approaches, while different, suggest that there might be ways in which healthy eating is relevant to multiculturalist thinking. In very general terms, we might have a multiculturalism-based concern that healthy eating efforts do not always respect/accommodate cultural difference.

For example, following Taylor we could argue that when it comes to eating, as in other areas of life and other aspects of our culture, we are embedded in our cultural, ethnic, or religious community. This community's eating habits shape us, and we have a normative obligation towards the other members of our community to sustain and preserve them. Furthermore, by non-recognizing or misrecognizing our culturally embedded eating practices, a state may cause us significant harm. This may happen, e.g., if the state imposes upon us healthy eating efforts that target foods central to our culture's eating practices, by neglecting their cultural relevance and decontextualizing them from our overall diets (which may be overall healthy diets despite the presence of specific foods that are, e.g., high in sugar, fat, or salt) (e.g. Davies 2013).

When it comes to Kymlicka's version of the argument, experiences of culturally significant food practices are experiences that are valuable to individuals because they are part of the cultural context that provides them with options for their exercise of individual autonomy. Crucially, for Kymlicka, the problem is that members of cultural minorities are at a disadvantage when it comes to access to their cultural contexts. According to this 'luck egalitarian' view, which considers any inequalities one is not responsible for unjust, members of cultural minorities should therefore be compensated, through the provision of group-differentiated rights. Healthy eating can be affected by these dynamics. If the state where I live does not protect or respect my culture's eating practices, or the conceptions of health and/or eating central to it (which may be different from those of the majority), I will be at a disadvantage in accessing my culturally related healthy eating practices. This may happen, e.g., if a state does not provide children of Muslim families with healthy eating options that comply with halal guidelines in school canteens.

But multiculturalism also has other implications. Liberal states often claim to be impartial and neutral in their laws and institutions. When it comes to healthy eating interventions, one might argue that these apply to all citizens equally and aim to promote a neutral goal, health, that all citizens can value despite their different cultural identities. Yet the impartiality and neutrality of liberal societies are often only apparent. When it comes to choosing an official 'neutral' language, e.g., '[a]rguments for civic neutrality with respect to . . . language rights equate and elide civic culture with what is, in effect, no more than a majoritarian form of linguistic nationalism' (May 2003, p. 138). Similarly, even when a state is formally secular, specific religious foundations may still affect its laws, public holidays, etc. All of this, according to some multiculturalist theorists, may require policies such as minority language rights or various forms of plural religious establishment (e.g. Modood 2013). Likewise, when it comes to healthy eating, the alleged impartiality and neutrality of such interventions may often presuppose biased cultural, religious, or even linguistic foundations, e.g. biased and culturally loaded conceptions of health or approaches to eating that reflect only the interests of the majority. This may require granting cultural minorities special rights to manage their own healthy eating interventions or pluralizing public understandings of healthy eating to incorporate those of minorities, so that no uniform approach to healthy eating is imposed upon all citizens.

But what measures, specifically, can a state implement in order to protect and promote people's access to their culture and the related healthy eating practices? Kymlicka (1995) provides a helpful categorization of three types of group-differentiated rights.

First, he argues that minorities, and especially indigenous groups and national minorities, should be granted self-government rights via such diverse institutional measures as federalism, reservations for Indigenous Americans (in North America), and Indigenous Protected Areas (in Australia), as well as control over health, education, language policy, veto rights over land, resources, etc. These rights resemble those invoked by advocates of food sovereignty, and may include specific control over healthy eating efforts.

Second, a multiculturalist state should promote what Kymlicka calls 'polyethnic rights', helping immigrants to integrate into the broader society. Polyethnic rights include state support for cultural activities and linguistic/educational programmes (bilingual education, faith schools, etc.). These may include food festivals and other activities promoting knowledge of that culture's approach to healthy eating. A further category of polyethnic rights concerns exemptions from existing laws, including, e.g., exemptions from animal-slaughtering laws for Muslim and Jewish people who consume halal and kosher meat. Other types of exemptions concern dress (e.g. Sikhs), military service (e.g. Quakers, Ultra-Orthodox Jews), and mandatory education (e.g. the Amish). When it comes to healthy eating, one could imagine measures similar to the halal and kosher exemptions, e.g. measures that exempt members of certain cultural or religious minorities from certain healthy eating efforts if these are in conflict with their cultural or religious beliefs.

Finally, there are special representation rights such as proportional representation and more inclusive political parties, affirmative action, guaranteed representation, separate electoral rolls (e.g. for Māori people in New Zealand), and affirmative gerrymandering. These may also be relevant to healthy eating efforts in the sense that having greater representation in key institutions may allow members of cultural minorities to have greater influence on policy decisions in this area, especially when such decisions may risk being in conflict with their culturally distinctive healthy eating practises.

Multiculturalism is, of course, not immune to criticisms. According to some, e.g., multiculturalism is an inappropriate response to the fact of cultural diversity, since members of cultural minorities should bear the (potentially burdensome) consequences of their cultural practices and beliefs, including the limits these may impose on the opportunities they can enjoy (Barry 2001). In response, it has been argued that if the costs of taking up an opportunity are unreasonable for an individual due to their minority cultural background, we cannot ask that person to (fully) bear those burdens (e.g. Miller 2002). Healthy eating efforts may not be culturally inclusive—e.g. they may involve subsidizing or promoting healthy versions of a dominant cuisine but not of minority cuisines, thus not being culturally appropriate for some groups. If, say, healthy eating options in schools or workplaces are provided only in non-halal or non-kosher versions, then if I am Muslim or Jewish the cost for me to enjoy the opportunity for healthy eating (and, indirectly, educational and job opportunities that result from being healthy) may be too high.

But what if the problem were not that different groups embrace different forms of healthy eating but, rather, that some cultural groups have norms and practices that strongly support healthy eating, and other cultural groups do not? For example, different groups may have different norms about body size, different norms about the importance of healthy eating, different norms about which foods are socially normative (e.g. is drinking sugary drinks normative or stigmatized?), and different culinary practices. Here it seems that the aforementioned idea of pluralizing access to opportunities might be helpful. In these cases, the desirable policy response may not be to impose one set of healthy eating-supportive norms and practices upon all groups but rather to promote good enough healthy eating amongst all groups while also recognizing that that there may be a plurality of pathways to well-being in different groups, e.g. different conceptions of health and well-being, some of which assign more priority to health as the absence of disease than others. Therefore, healthy eating efforts for some groups should emphasize not only eating in ways that reduce disease risk, but also eating in ways that promote health as they understand it.

2.6. Healthy eating efforts, perfectionism, and neutrality

The idea of state neutrality is central to much contemporary liberal political philosophy, and especially to theories of political liberalism. The central tenet of state neutrality is that the state ought not to adopt political perfectionism; i.e. it ought not to legislate on the basis of one or more controversial conceptions of the good, i.e. contentious views on how citizens ought to lead their lives. But what, more specifically, is state neutrality?

There are normally two main ways of understanding state neutrality. On the one hand, one may refer to *neutrality of consequences*. This demands that the state should not legislate in ways that have the effect of privileging one or a few conceptions of the good, allowing it/them to flourish more than others. For example, a state may not endorse a particular religion over others if doing so results in that religion gaining more adherents than others (or than non-religious conceptions of the good). The obvious problem with this view is that it is virtually impossible to foresee all the effects of state laws and policies or to make all the adjustments necessary to rectify any unequal effects that may arise along the way. For this reason, neutrality of consequences is normally rejected as a suitable conception of state neutrality (Merrill 2014).

The other main understanding of state neutrality, and the one that we embrace, is the idea of neutrality of aims, or *neutrality of justifications*. While the two are sometimes treated separately, they in fact present very similar features and, for our purposes here, they can be discussed interchangeably. For this reason, we will simply refer to 'neutrality of justifications' from now onwards. The core tenet of neutrality of justifications is the idea that while many (perhaps most) state laws inevitably have the *effect* of privileging one or a few conceptions of the good over others, this is not morally problematic as long as the rationale for the state to implement such laws is neutral; i.e. it does not appeal to any particular conception of the good. The most prominent version of this argument is the one endorsed by those liberals who defend the idea of 'public reason' (Gaus 2011; Larmore 1996; Quong 2011; Rawls 2005a). Public reason is the view that state laws and policies can legitimately be implemented only if they are justified on the basis of reasons that are public, i.e. reasons that all citizens can accept at some level of idealization despite their different conceptions of the good. The idea of public reason is based on two key assumptions.

First, contemporary liberal societies are fundamentally diverse. They are characterized by the fact of reasonable pluralism or disagreement (Rawls 2005a). This is pluralism or disagreement among persons who are 'ready to propose principles and standards as fair terms of cooperation and to abide by them willingly, given the assurance that others will likewise do so' (Rawls 2005a, p. 49), and who accept the 'burdens of judgment', i.e. 'the many hazards involved in the correct (and conscientious) exercise of our powers of reason and judgment in the ordinary course of political life' (Rawls 2005a, p. 56). These include, e.g., the complexity of empirical evidence, the fact that concepts are vague, and the different ways in which individuals weigh opposing considerations regarding empirical and moral issues.

Second, compelling citizens to obey political rules based on reasons they cannot accept entails failing to treat them as free and equal persons, i.e. to recognize that '[e]ach of us is free in the sense of not being naturally subject to any other person's moral or political authority, and [that] we are equally situated with respect to this freedom from the natural authority of others'

(Quong 2018). In order to treat other citizens as free and equal, in view of the fact of reasonable disagreement, we need to provide them with a justification as to why they should obey political rules. Justifications for political rules should be based on reasons that all citizens could accept at some level of idealization.

Public reason excludes from public justification controversial reasons such as those provided by religious, ethical, and philosophical doctrines not shared by all citizens in contemporary diverse societies. For example, a law cannot be justified by appealing to reasons grounded in Catholicism or Islam, as Hindus or atheists (amongst others) would not accept such reasons, and vice versa. In other words, such reasons are not *public* reasons. Conversely, according to political liberals, some reasons are public and therefore acceptable by all citizens in spite of reasonable disagreement. These include, e.g., reasons referring to basic rights and liberties (e.g. freedom of thought and conscience, freedom of religion, freedom of association, etc.) as well as reasons referring to equality of opportunity and the common good (Rawls 2005a, pp. 223–24). These political values belong to the public political culture of liberal democratic societies, and political rules are publicly justified if their aim is to protect and promote these values. Furthermore, public reason also includes 'the methods and conclusions of science when these are not controversial' (p. 224) as well as 'plain truths now widely accepted, or available, to citizens generally' (p. 224) and 'presently accepted general beliefs and forms of reasoning found in common sense' (p. 224).

The debate on public reason is especially relevant to healthy eating efforts. Indeed in this book, and especially from Chapter 5 onwards, we will focus on the following question: when, if ever, are healthy eating efforts, i.e. policies, programmes, and interventions aimed at promoting healthier eating, publicly justified and consistent with the idea of public reason? Our rationale for asking this question, and for adopting public reason as a framework, is the following. We believe that healthy eating efforts are both necessary and desirable in contemporary liberal societies. However, we also believe that the design of such efforts should be accompanied by a greater acknowledgement of the complex moral issues that surround them than is currently the case. Public reason offers a promising framework for analysing such issues.

First, public reason takes into account the reasonable pluralism or disagreement that characterizes contemporary liberal societies. The issue of reasonable pluralism or disagreement, we believe, is especially relevant to the analysis of healthy eating efforts. People in liberal democratic societies conceive of health and eating in diverse ways and assign various forms of value and disvalue to different dietary patterns, healthy and unhealthy. This fact ought to become more central to the normative assessment of healthy eating efforts.

Second, public reason can help make sense of the complex moral universe that surrounds healthy eating efforts. Such efforts involve empirical, epistemic, and moral considerations that are deeply interrelated. It is therefore not sufficient to assess them based on the extent to which they promote a specific moral value such as liberty or equality. Instead, multiple moral values can be promoted or hindered by such efforts, and should be reckoned with. Furthermore, different empirical and epistemic assumptions often underlie healthy eating efforts, e.g. those concerning the causal relationship between eating and health (or lack thereof). Sometimes, we will see, the empirical evidence in this area is weak or subject to scientific controversy. Nevertheless, we will argue, it may still be justifiable to implement healthy eating efforts if certain conditions are in place. The key point, for now, is that public reason (or, more specifically, the conception of public reason that we will defend in this book—'accessibility') can help us to take into account all these various empirical, epistemic, and moral issues within a unified framework.

2.7. Healthy eating efforts and political legitimacy

The last theme that we would like to examine in this chapter is the idea of political legitimacy, another central concept in political philosophy. Political legitimacy can be understood in both an empirical and a normative sense. The former refers to the *beliefs* that people in a society have regarding the government's right to impose laws upon them, and their duty to obey them. Empirical political legitimacy is therefore a sociological concept, perhaps best instantiated by the work of Max Weber ([1918] 1991, 1964), who famously distinguished between three sources of political legitimacy or authority: tradition, charisma, and the rule of law.

However, political philosophers are mainly concerned with *normative* political legitimacy. This is not grounded in people's beliefs but rather in some moral standard based on which the exercise of state power can be considered more or less rightful. Normative political legitimacy is closely related to the ideas of public justification and public reason that we introduced in the previous section, and which are central to the remainder of the book.

More specifically, public reason is one of many potential sources of political legitimacy. According to this view, in societies characterized by reasonable disagreement, state power can be legitimately exercised only if political rules (e.g. laws and policies) are justified by appealing to public reasons. The connection between normative political legitimacy and public reason is best captured by Rawls' (2005, p. 137) liberal principle of legitimacy, according to which

> [o]ur exercise of political power is fully proper only when it is exercised in accordance with a constitution the essentials of which all citizens as free and equal may reasonably be expected to endorse in the light of principles and ideals acceptable to their common human reason.[6]

However, public reason is only one of many possible sources of political legitimacy. An alternative conception of political legitimacy, and one which is the forebear of public reason, is grounded in the idea of consent. According to this view, political power is legitimately exercised only when those subject to it have consented to it (Locke 1980; Nozick 1974; Simmons 2001). This consent can be expressed (i.e. explicitly provided, e.g. verbally or in writing), tacit (i.e. it can be implied from people's actions and behaviour), or, according to some, even hypothetical (i.e. as the consent that people *would give* to political rules under certain ideal conditions) (Peter 2017). Hypothetical consent is the type of consent that is most closely related to public reason since the latter, we have seen, involves providing reasons for political rules that most if not all citizens *would accept* at some level of idealization.

A further conception of political legitimacy is consequentialist in nature. According to this view, state power is legitimately exercised only when it produces beneficial outcomes (Binmore 2000). More specifically, according to a specific and influential strand of consequentialism called utilitarianism, political power is legitimate only when it contributes to society's happiness (Bentham [1789] 1907). A common criticism of utilitarianism is that it may justify the infringement of some people's rights and liberties if this contributes to increasing happiness overall within society. However, other conceptions of utilitarianism try to reconcile the promotion of the greatest good with the protection of individual rights and liberties. According to John

---

[6] As we will explain in Chapter 6, we embrace a more expansive account of the scope of public reason than Rawls does and believe that public reason applies to all legislation rather than only to constitutional essentials and matters of basic justice.

Stuart Mill ([1859] 2006, p. 17), e.g., happiness is 'grounded on the permanent interests of man as a progressive being'. This involves the exercise of our intellectual and deliberative faculties, which is possible only if we enjoy a significant degree of freedom from the interference of the state and other citizens. Furthermore, 'rule utilitarians' (e.g. Hooker 2000) argue that society's greatest good is best promoted by following rules, including laws that protect individual rights and liberties.

Finally, another important source of political legitimacy is democracy, a concept that we examined in a previous section. Here we can distinguish between procedural and epistemic conceptions of democratic legitimacy. The former is the view that the exercise of state power is legitimate as long as it results from democratic procedures, independently from the outcomes these produce (e.g. Peter 2008). As we have already seen when considering the difference between aggregative and deliberative democracy, democratic procedures may include free and fair elections as well as forums and processes through which citizens engage in democratic deliberation. The epistemic conception is instead the view that democratic procedures contribute to political legitimacy only if they produce decisions that correspond to or approximate certain ideal outcomes (Estlund 2008).

What are the implications of our discussion of political legitimacy for healthy eating policy? In the remainder of the book, we will consider in detail two of these conceptions. One is, of course, the public justification view, which is central to our main argument. The other is the Millian conception, which combines utilitarian and liberal elements, and which we examine in the next chapter. We will employ both conceptions to evaluate when and under which conditions healthy eating efforts may be politically legitimate, i.e. rightfully imposed by the state on its citizens. However, there is a sense in which elements of the other conceptions too are also relevant to our account of healthy eating policy. For example, public justification is linked to consent, and the latter can play an important role in the kinds of consultation processes that we defend in Chapter 7. Likewise, deliberative forums for the discussion of healthy eating policy, which we also defend in that chapter, combine elements of procedural democratic legitimacy and public justification.

Furthermore, one of the ideas that underlies our analysis in this book is that publicly justified healthy eating efforts are not only more respectful of citizens' free and equal status—a key aspect of public reason—but also ultimately better and likely more effective than those that lack public justification. This is because they are grounded in a fuller evidence base and greater awareness of the potential social economic, and other effects that their implementation may have for different groups of people (two aspects of public reason that we examine in Chapters 6 and 7). In this way, our analysis has a point of overlap with the epistemic conception of democratic legitimacy: we consider the outcomes produced by a process of public justification and public reasoning—in this case, more effective healthy eating efforts—to be important criteria when fashioning such a process.

In sum, the foregoing overview of political legitimacy and, more generally, the analysis conducted in this chapter can help us and the reader to better situate our public reason approach to healthy eating policy within the context of key concepts, theories, and debates in normative political philosophy.

3

Healthy Eating Efforts and
Millian Liberalism

3.1. Introduction

In this chapter we illustrate the implications of John Stuart Mill's liberalism
for healthy eating efforts. We especially focus on the arguments advanced
by Mill ([1859] 2006) in his classic essay *On Liberty*. There are a number of
reasons why it is worth spending some time in this book applying Mill's liberal philosophy to the case of healthy eating policy.

First, Mill is one of the main exponents of *perfectionist liberalism*, which
is centred around the value of individual autonomy and emphasizes the
need for the state to legislate in ways that promote its citizens' autonomous
flourishing in all aspects of their lives. A focus on perfectionist liberalism in
relation to healthy eating will help the reader understand better the non-per-
fectionist political approach that we will adopt in the remainder of the book,
which is epitomized by the work of John Rawls. Second, efforts targeting
unhealthy dietary patterns are often accused of being strongly paternalistic,
and Mill is normally considered the archetype of a liberal anti-paternalist
thinker (e.g. see Saunders 2013). Mill's ideas are often invoked by those who
oppose state paternalism (Powers et al. 2012), both within and outside ac-
ademia, including those who reject policies limiting the sale of unhealthy
foods.[1] To cite just one recent example, already mentioned in Chapter 1,
when a few years ago NYC former mayor Michael Bloomberg proposed the
ban of large-size sugary drinks, Marty Markowitz, the borough president
of Brooklyn, appealed to Mill's alleged anti-paternalism when making his
case against the measure (which was eventually approved by the NYC Board

---

[1] As we already explained in Chapter 1, we use 'unhealthy foods' as shorthand to refer to foods that
are widely consumed at levels that pose health risks. 'Unhealthy foods' include, e.g. candy, sugary
beverages, and processed foods high in fat, sugar, or salt.

Healthy Eating Policy and Political Philosophy. Anne Barnhill and Matteo Bonotti, Oxford University Press. © Oxford
University Press 2022. DOI: 10.1093/oso/9780190937881.003.0004

of Health, though subsequently rejected by the courts) (Anonymous 2012c, 2014). [2]

Third, due to their central place in the history of liberalism, Mill's views have already been invoked by various authors in relation to other health policy areas, including alcohol minimum pricing (Saunders 2013) and genetically modified food (Holtug 2001). Discussing the implications of Mill's theory for healthy eating policy therefore seems to be a natural extension of this body of literature. Finally, Mill's ([1859] 2006) account in the essay *On Liberty* offers a systematic normative framework for evaluating different types of healthy eating efforts, including nutrition fact labels, food advertising and 'fat taxes'.

Nevertheless, Mill's almost exclusive concern for liberty implies that a Millian assessment of healthy eating efforts displays significant limits. As we explained in the previous chapter, one of the main ethical issues surrounding such efforts concerns the complex trade-offs that citizens face when engaging in (un)healthy eating, trade-offs that policymakers should take into account when designing and implementing healthy eating efforts. By foregrounding individual liberty, a Millian approach inevitably overlooks other important dimensions of (un)healthy eating and therefore cannot provide a satisfactory holistic framework for policymaking in this area.

Our analysis proceeds as follows. First, we assess whether and to what extent Mill's 'harm principle' justifies social and legal non-paternalistic penalties against people with unhealthy dietary patterns who are guilty of other-regarding harm. Second, we show that Mill's account warrants taxing unhealthy foods, thus restricting the freedom of both eaters Mill would have considered 'responsible' and those he would have considered 'irresponsible', and de facto justifying some degree of paternalism in the area of healthy eating policy. Finally, we show that Mill's account warrants some restrictions on food advertising and justifies various forms of food labelling.

3.2. Mill's 'harm principle'

The central thread of Mill's ([1859] 2006, p. 16) essay *On Liberty* is what is known as the 'harm principle', i.e. the idea

---

[2] We set aside, in this chapter, a comprehensive assessment of the contemporary scholarly debates on paternalism (e.g. see Arneson 1980, 2005; Coons and Weber 2014; De Marneffe 2006; Dworkin 1997; Feinberg 1971; Shiffrin 2000; Sunstein and Thaler 2003). We will engage with some of those broader debates in Chapter 3.

that the sole end for which mankind are warranted, individually or collectively, in interfering with the liberty of action of any of their number . . . against his will, is to prevent harm to others. His own good, either physical or moral, is not a sufficient warrant.

Mill's harm principle is aimed at protecting 'the appropriate region of human liberty' (p. 18) from the unwarranted interference of state and/or society. That region, Mill argues, comprises 'the inward domain of consciousness . . . liberty of tastes and pursuits . . . [and] the liberty . . . of combination between individuals' (pp. 18–19).

While the debate on Mill's conception of harm is vast and characterized by internal disagreements (e.g. Rees 1960; Riley 1991, 1998, pp. 75–76, 98–99), a few aspects of it are unequivocal and find broad support amongst scholars. First, for Mill ([1859] 2006, pp. 61–63) mere offence is not harm. Second, interference with an individual's liberty is warranted not only when there is actual harm but also '[w]henever . . . there is . . . a definite risk of damage, either to an individual or to the public' (p. 93). This is important when considering the potential harmful consequences (to others) of unhealthy dietary patterns, as we will show later in the chapter. Third, for Mill harm is a necessary but not sufficient condition for interfering with an individual's freedom. Indeed, even in the case of some other-regarding harms, Mill argues, interference is not warranted 'either because it is a kind of case in which he is on the whole likely to act better, when left to his own discretion . . . or because the attempt to exercise control would produce other evils, greater than those which it would prevent' (p. 18).[3]

Fourth, the distinction between 'self-regarding' and 'other-regarding' conduct, which is central to Mill's essay, is especially problematic and indeed has been the object of an intense debate amongst Mill's critics (e.g. see Rees 1960; Riley 1998, pp. 99ff.). The main problem, according to many, is that any self-regarding act and, most importantly, any self-regarding harm is likely to have consequences upon other individuals. Mill ([1859] 2006, p. 92, emphasis added), however, is not unaware of this issue and argues that only when, due to self-harming conduct, 'a person is led to violate *a distinct and assignable obligation* to any other person or persons, the case is taken out of the self-regarding

---

[3] Mill ([1859] 2006, p. 107) provides the example of the harm and suffering that someone who 'succeeds in an overcrowded profession, or in a competitive examination' may cause upon losing competitors. According to Mill, this kind of 'harm' does not warrant interference with individual liberty unless 'means of success have been employed which it is contrary to the general interest to permit—namely, fraud or treachery, and force' (p. 107).

class, and becomes amenable to moral disapprobation in the proper sense of the term'. Shortly thereafter, he highlights that 'when a person disables himself, by conduct purely self-regarding, from the performance of *some definite duty incumbent on him to the public*, he is guilty of a social offence. No person ought to be punished simply for being drunk; but a soldier or a policeman should be punished for being drunk on duty' (pp. 92–93, emphasis added). What renders actions harmful, therefore, is for Mill the breach of specific obligations and duties we have towards other people. As J. C. Rees (1960, p. 119) observes, for Mill harm occurs not merely when someone's actions affect others (something which is inevitable for most of people's actions) but when they affect other people's interests, and 'interests . . . depend for their existence on social recognition and are closely connected with prevailing standards about the sort of behaviour a man can legitimately expect from others'.

Fifth, and finally, Mill's harm principle articulates his rejection of state paternalism. An individual's 'own good, either physical or moral, is not a sufficient warrant', we have seen, for 'interfering with the liberty or action' of that individual (Mill [1859] 2006, p. 16). But how exactly should paternalism be understood? In this chapter we follow Gerald Dworkin (1997, p. 62, emphasis added) in defining paternalism as 'the interference with a person's liberty of action justified by *reasons* referring exclusively to the welfare, good, happiness, needs, interests or values of the person being coerced'. The emphasis, therefore, should be on the *reasons* presented by legislators to justify laws and policies. Dworkin rightly points out that while any law or policy can in principle be justified on different grounds, paternalistic measures are only those which, even when non-paternalistic arguments are also available, are justified by appealing to an agent's own good and aim to protect her from purely self-regarding harm. While considering Dworkin's definition of paternalism especially useful for the scope of our present discussion in this chapter, we are aware that, due to disagreement about the nature of paternalism, it is not the only (or, for some, the best) one.[4]

Does Mill's 'harm principle' justify social and legal non-paternalistic penalties against people with unhealthy dietary patterns who are guilty of other-regarding harm? If so, to what extent? And does Mill's account also justify paternalistic measures? We turn to those questions in the following sections.

---

[4] We will offer a more thorough analysis of paternalism in Chapter 4, where we will also endorse a different definition of paternalism, i.e. that provided by Jonathan Quong (2011).

3.3. Unhealthy dietary patterns and harm to others: Harm as a necessary but not sufficient condition for intervention

Mill's rejection of paternalism, expressed by the harm principle, makes it morally unacceptable for the state to implement legislation prohibiting or restricting the consumption of unhealthy foods in order to promote the health of the consumers themselves and prevent them from incurring self-regarding harm, as we discuss later. In light of this, one might suggest a work-around: an unhealthy dietary pattern is other-regarding harmful conduct, because it imposes costs on other people besides the eater herself. It is therefore necessary to assess whether and under what circumstances unhealthy eating can be considered other-regarding harmful conduct, thus falling outside the scope of the harm principle. This is what we intend to do in this and the following sections.

It is often argued that drinking alcohol and smoking are instances of other-regarding harmful conduct. Drinking, as Mill himself highlights, can potentially (though not necessarily) lead to harmful other-regarding conduct. 'The making himself drunk, in a person whom drunkenness excites to do harm to others', Mill ([1859] 2006, p. 110) argues, 'is a crime against others'. Even more clearly, smoking can often harm other people directly (i.e. through second-hand smoke). This was one of the central arguments behind the smoking bans implemented in many countries over the past two decades, and was the central argument for smoking bans in public places in the US (Bayer 2007).[5] It is difficult to argue, however, that unhealthy eating can have the same harmful effects on others.

But some researchers have tried to make the case. Empirical research has shown, for example, that weight gain (e.g. due to unhealthy dietary patterns) can be 'contagious' under certain family and social conditions (e.g. Christakis and Fowler 2007). Furthermore, food aromas (e.g. in shopping malls) can attract people and induce them to consume unhealthy foods 'because the sensory information goes to the lower, primitive or reactive parts of the brains before they ever get to the higher, reasoning part' (McKenzie 2012, pp. 168–69).

Each of these arguments deserves to be critically assessed. At first glance, the claim that weight gain is contagious may seem to stretch the meaning

---

[5] Observers of public health, however, have questioned whether these arguments might be disingenuous (Bayer 2007; Colgrove and Bayer 2005); what might actually animate these efforts is the desire to improve people's lives by making them healthier, but this intention is masked in order to preempt the charge of paternalism.

of 'contagious' beyond recognition—as if mere exposure to other people's dietary patterns or weight causes it—and to underestimate the importance of voluntary choice in responding to social conditions. Yet we should be careful in endorsing this conclusion. One's food choices can have significant effects upon other people's eating habits. After all eating, we saw in Chapter 1, is often also a social activity. Consider, e.g., the degree of social conditioning that especially characterizes the internal life of families. Children are especially likely to be socialized into the eating habits of their parents. If the latter have an unhealthy dietary pattern, then this is likely both to have negative effects on their children's health (see Merry 2012) and, more generally, to influence the children's future dietary patterns. Should the state therefore be allowed to intervene in order to regulate the eating habits of families?

Here, it should be noted, the question is not simply whether the state should be allowed to interfere *directly* with children's dietary patterns in order to prevent them from developing diet-related illness. Mill ([1859] 2006, p. 16) would not have problems with this kind of intervention as the harm principle does not apply to 'children, or . . . young persons below the age which the law may fix as that of manhood or womanhood'. This would justify, e.g., such measures as restricting the sale of unhealthy foods to children in school canteens and establishing a minimum age for buying such foods in shops, cafes, and restaurants.

The more problematic question, however, is whether the state should also interfere *indirectly* with children's dietary patterns, i.e. by interfering with the internal life of those families in which children have diet-related illness, or risk factors for diet-related illness, due to the family eating habits. A positive answer to this question would raise the spectre of an all-encompassing interventionist state, which sits very uneasily with Mill's views. Justifying this kind of intervention could also potentially justify other kinds of interference with families' internal lives, in order to address other activities and situations that can potentially harm children. By following the same line of argument, one could justify not only interference with family eating habits but also interference with the choices of those families where there are 'parents who are divorced, who smoke, whose children play outside without sunscreen, whose children watch several hours of television a day, whose children attend conservative religious schools, whose children play contact sports' (Merry 2012, p. 5). All these activities and situations can potentially cause harm to children and affect their physical and/or psychological health.

We have seen that the harm principle, however, is a necessary but not sufficient condition for interfering with the liberty of others, and that sometimes 'the attempt to exercise control [i.e. in this case, to regulate extensively the internal life of families] would produce other evils, greater than those which it would prevent' (Mill [1859] 2006, p. 18). When it comes to enforcing healthy eating habits within families, these side effects might include the disruption of a harmonious family life or of parents' ability to dedicate more time and resources to other activities with their children that we illustrated in Chapter 1. We therefore doubt that Mill would have justified *systematic* state interference with the internal life of families. But it remains an open question whether Mill would have accepted *certain limited kinds of interference*, i.e. those for which the attempt to exercise control does not produce greater evils than those it prevents.

A similar conclusion can be made regarding the second example. Even if (and it is a big 'if') it could be shown that food aromas often compel or strongly encourage individuals to consume certain (unhealthy) foods (i.e. through a kind of irrational compulsion/addiction), and that therefore those who eat (or cook) these foods in public are somehow harming others, we should ask whether this would warrant restrictions and controls from a Millian perspective. These restrictions, it should be noted, would need to be quite radical, ranging from the prohibition of eating such foods in certain public places to the obligation for 'unhealthy eateries' located in crowded areas (e.g. shopping malls) to serve their customers behind tightly closed doors. It seems likely that these kinds of interventions would cause more harm than they would prevent, and therefore would be impermissible from the perspective of Mill's harm principle.

3.4. Unhealthy dietary patterns and harm to others: Specific duties to others

There are, however, cases in which unhealthy dietary patterns may lead to the infringement of specific duties and obligations we have towards other people, and in which state intervention would probably not cause more harm than it would prevent. In such cases, state interference may be justified on Millian grounds. For example, Mill ([1859] 2006, pp. 92–93) highlights, '[n]o person ought to be punished simply for being drunk; but a soldier or a policeman should be punished for being drunk on duty'. The soldier and policeman, in

Mill's example, have voluntarily undertaken specific obligations[6] towards the public (e.g. the taxpayer) and their employer (e.g. the state), but drunkenness prevents them from fulfilling them. This is what renders their conduct morally condemnable and justifies punishing them.

If we apply this line of argument to the issue of unhealthy dietary patterns, Mill's views can be used to justify, e.g., fining athletes who have unhealthy dietary patterns and, as a consequence, gain weight or become affected by other diet-related health problems (coronary disease, high blood pressure, diabetes, etc.). It is especially important for (most) athletes to be healthy and keep their weight low in order to fulfil the duties they have voluntarily undertaken towards their employer, as well as towards supporters, sponsors, etc. According to this line of argument, therefore, Mill's account would seem to permit, e.g., the fines that football club West Ham imposed upon football player Benni McCarthy for being overweight during the 2010–11 season (Edwards 2010). Since McCarthy had voluntarily undertaken contractual obligations towards his team and committed to providing it with his football services, and on the assumption that not being overweight is a crucial condition for the latter, his club was morally entitled to fine him from a Millian perspective.

Similarly, more demanding fitness tests for police officers, and penalties for those of them who are overweight (e.g. Anonymous 2012b), are justifiable in Millian terms if the rationale is to ensure that police officers are able to perform their job properly. In more general terms, whenever the discharge of a voluntarily undertaken obligation is jeopardized by one's diet-related illness and/or by being overweight, and these are a consequence of unhealthy dietary patterns (rather than of an underlying health condition, genetic factors, etc.), then moral reprehension and penalties (fines, suspension, etc.) are justifiable in Millian terms. If, however, not being overweight is not essential for performing one's job, being penalized for being overweight due to one's unhealthy dietary patterns would clearly be an instance of discrimination, unjustifiable from a Millian perspective.

Mill ([1859] 2006, p. 92) also argues that

[i]f . . . a man, through intemperance or extravagance, becomes unable to pay his debts, or, having undertaken the moral responsibility of a family,

---

[6] We set aside here the problems concerning the moral bindingness of obligations which have not been voluntarily undertaken. Please also note that we use the terms 'duty' and 'obligation' interchangeably.

becomes from the same cause incapable of supporting or educating them, he is deservedly reprobated, and might be justly punished; but it is for the breach of duty to his family or creditors, not for the extravagance.

Mill reinforces this point by arguing that

if, either from idleness or from any other avoidable cause, a man fails to perform his legal duties to others, as for instance to support his children, it is no tyranny to force him to fulfil that obligation, by compulsory labour, if no other means are available. (p. 111)

Like in the cases of the drunk policeman and soldier and of the overweight footballer, these examples point to the moral blameworthiness of rendering oneself unable to fulfil one's voluntarily undertaken duties, i.e. towards one's family or one's creditors. But it may be more difficult, in these cases, to understand what kinds of measures Mill would have endorsed in order to punish individuals guilty of 'food intemperance', even if we can show that their dietary pattern causes the condition that incapacitates them. Mill mentions 'compulsory labour', but the problem is that the negligent eater (like the negligent drinker or smoker) may often be unable to perform *any* labour (e.g. due to some disabling condition) and therefore fulfil their obligations (e.g. financial ones) towards their creditors or family. How can society then compel the (as Mill might put it) 'negligent' or 'irresponsible' eater to fulfil their obligations in these cases?

It should be remembered here that for Mill ([1859] 2006, p. 18) harmful actions towards others are not morally condemnable when they are performed 'with their free, voluntary, and undeceived consent and participation'. This implies that the state should not compel 'negligent' or 'irresponsible' eaters to fulfil their obligations, if those whose interests are being damaged do not demand that. But it may also imply that we have a right to demand of others that our interests not be damaged by their negligent actions. What concretely follows from this? One implication is that lenders, e.g., could be given the right (but not the duty) to attach compulsory insurance policies to the loans they offer to customers, as well as to inspect borrowers' health conditions (including their weight, lifestyle, and any food-related illnesses) and adjust the insurance premiums accordingly. Moreover, in order to minimize the costs for 'responsible' eaters and any risk of abuse, once a loan has been fully paid back, all the insurance premiums could be returned to the borrower (e.g. as in the case of 'return of premium' life insurance policies). This would not defeat the scope of these insurance policies which, it should be made clear, is to prevent lenders from incurring a financial loss, not to increase their profits.[7]

What about the man who 'through intemperance or extravagance . . . having undertaken the moral responsibility of a family, becomes from the same cause incapable of supporting or educating them' (Mill [1859] 2006, p. 92)? This is a more sensitive matter, and state interventions to ensure that obligations are fulfilled should therefore be more cautious. Yet it could still be argued that, from a Millian perspective, spouses should have the right not only to morally condemn their negligent partners but also to demand material (e.g. financial) guarantees from them if they fail (or there is a significant risk that they may fail) to fulfil their obligations due to their dietary patterns. Mill, we have seen, even allows the use of 'compulsory labour' in these instances. His account may therefore also justify a spouse's right (protected and enforced by the state) to legally oblige their partner to take out a life or critical illness insurance policy, when there are significant grounds to believe that their dietary patterns may lead to death or seriously incapacitate them in the future.

These measures, of course, might be open to abuse. However, as in the case of insurance policies imposed upon borrowers, also in this instance the 'return of premiums' formula could be adopted in order to minimize the risk of misuse against spouses who are healthy eaters. Moreover, special institutions may be established in order to monitor controversial cases, e.g. when one spouse refuses to take out an insurance policy upon the partner's request. Regardless of the specific details of these measures, and the practical difficulties they might involve, they would be compatible with Mill's account as long as they were aimed at preventing harm to those individuals (e.g. spouse, children) who depend on the person with an unhealthy dietary pattern. Moreover, these tailored measures would avoid imposing unfair burdens (e.g. in the form of a 'fat tax') upon healthier eaters and similarly unhealthy eaters who have not undertaken any voluntary commitments towards creditors, spouses, etc., and therefore can harm only themselves.

This section has argued that Mill would have supported measures penalizing unhealthy dietary patterns when the latter prevent people from

---

[7] In fact, however, these insurance policies would also still provide an additional benefit for lenders, i.e. in the form of available funds to be invested elsewhere while waiting for the loan to be fully repaid.

fulfilling role-specific duties towards others. Arguably, Mill would have also supported moral disapproval directed toward such people. However, holding people accountable for their eating in these ways may seem unfair, or otherwise inappropriate. As we pointed out in the previous chapters, people may have circumscribed control over their eating, given the social, psychological, physiological, and environmental influences on eating behaviour, and it is unfair to hold people accountable for behaviour that they do not sufficiently control.[8] This therefore undermines, or at least qualifies, this line of argument in Mill's account.

It is possible that Mill himself would agree with this objection. Plausibly Mill would think that compulsion and penalties are appropriate only if the cause is under the person's control—recall his words that

> if either from idleness *or from any other avoidable cause*, a man fails to perform his legal duties to others, as for instance to support his children, it is no tyranny to force him to fulfil that obligation, by compulsory labour, if no other means are available. (Mill [1859] 2006, p. 111, emphasis added)

The key question, then, is whether dietary patterns are avoidable in the relevant sense.

3.5. Unhealthy dietary patterns and harm to others: Public healthcare costs

There is a further sense in which, according to some, unhealthy dietary patterns can be considered a conduct that harms others. Individuals whose behaviour significantly increases their health and safety risks (e.g. having a dietary pattern that poses a significant risk of diet-related illness, smoking, riding a motorcycle without a helmet, etc.), according to this view, run a risk of being a burden on state finances (e.g. because they may require extra healthcare, extra caretaking, and extra social support), and this constitutes a harm against people with safer and healthier behaviour who have to share that burden (e.g. see Jones and Bayer 2007, p. 211). This argument is not an idle theoretical possibility. As Colgrove and Bayer (2005, pp. 573–74) note, when motorcycle helmet laws were broadly adopted in the US in the 1960s

---

[8] See e.g. Dixon (2018).

and 1970s, they were objected to as paternalistic, and legal challenges were made. Court opinions upholding these laws 'sought to demonstrate that the social impact of private behavior provided ample warrant for legislative action' (p. 574)—in other words, the financial costs that motorcycle injury imposes on the public purse (including the costs of emergency responders, healthcare, as well as potentially disability and unemployment insurance) harm others, and therefore justify coercing motorcyclists into wearing a helmet. Thus motorcycle helmet laws are not paternalistic public health policies, despite initial appearances.

A number of responses can be provided to this argument that individual behaviour significantly increasing one's own risk of injury and disease constitutes a harm against other people. To start with, Mill ([1859] 2006, p. 93) himself observes that

> with regard to the merely contingent, or . . . constructive injury which a person causes to society, by conduct which neither violates any specific duty to the public, nor occasions perceptible hurt to any assignable individual except himself; the inconvenience is one which society can afford to bear, for the sake of the greater good of human freedom.

Society, Mill thinks, need not use coercive measures in these instances but rather should prevent certain 'costly' behaviours (e.g. dietary patterns that cause health problems) through other means, including 'all the powers of education . . . and . . . the natural penalties which cannot be prevented on those who incur the distaste or the contempt of those who know them' (pp. 93–94). Education to healthier eating through nutrition education programmes and messaging campaigns, therefore, would be welcomed by Mill. According to him, persuasion and advice (i.e. rather than compulsion) are entirely consistent with the harm principle.

Yet it is worth noting that Mill is not entirely clear about what a 'constructive injury' (as in the previous quote) precisely is, and how it differs from a real and damaging injury. In the *Principles of Political Economy*, e.g., Mill ([1848] 1965a) argues that members of the working class (and Mill especially blames men) who have many children contribute to a decrease of the wage rate, thus causing a real (and not merely 'constructive') injury to their fellows. He therefore argues that it would be justified to use social pressure in order to persuade working-class families to have only a limited number of children. Should social pressure not suffice, Mill even argues that 'there would be then an evident justification for converting the moral obligation against bringing children into the world who are a burthen to the community, into a legal one' (p. 372).

There are some similarities between this example and the case of eaters with dietary patterns that significantly increase the risk of diet-related illness. In both cases, certain individuals perform actions (i.e. have many children, have a certain dietary pattern) which in themselves may have insignificant effects but which, when performed by most people, are deleterious to other individuals and cause them a real injury (e.g. by reducing their wealth through lower wages or higher taxes). Mill ([1848] 1965a, p. 371) himself emphasizes 'the disgrace which naturally and inevitably attends on conduct by any one individual, which if pursued by a majority, everybody can see would be fatal'. Therefore, it is by no means clear that Mill would have rejected penalties against eaters who contribute to increasing a society's healthcare costs.

Yet, further considerations are required on this issue. As John Skorupski (2006, p. 46) points out, arguing that the financial burden imposed by 'irresponsible' citizens (he specifically refers to motorcyclists who do not wear a helmet, but his argument could also be extended to people with unhealthy dietary patterns) harms society 'dangerously stretches the notion of "harm"'. However, even if we grant, for the sake of argument, that imposing an increased financial burden upon the healthcare system *does* harm society, there are a number of possible replies to this point.

First, even if one's dietary pattern harms society (through increased healthcare costs), the same could also be argued of other potentially risky activities, such as 'driving, hiking, skiing, parasailing . . . biking, surfing . . . jaywalking' (McKenzie 2012, p. 231). Most activities individuals engage in carry certain risks (and potential healthcare costs), and this line of reasoning may easily lead to the conclusion that if we impose penalties upon 'irresponsible' eaters we should also penalize 'irresponsible' hikers, skiers, etc., for the additional financial burden they impose (or risk imposing) upon society. Therefore, this would just mean imposing some kinds of penalties on almost every individual, as almost everyone is probably engaged at some point in some (potentially) risky activity.

Furthermore, while some risky activities (e.g. jaywalking) are admittedly gratuitous, in the sense that they do not plausibly make the lives of those who engage in them better and more valuable, the same is not true of many other risky activities. Those who love skiing or hiking normally believe that the risks of injury deriving from their cherished activities are worth taking, and that abandoning those activities would render their lives less valuable. The same can also be said about dietary patterns that increase health risks, which can often have value for many individuals (e.g. Barnhill et al. 2014; Resnik 2010), as we explained in the previous chapters.

Given that many valuable human activities, including dietary patterns, are often carriers of important values for those who engage in them, it could be argued that this justifies having in place some kind of public healthcare system through which all members of society are collectively insured against the negative consequences that most human activities carry with them. As Skorupski (2006, p. 46) cogently highlights (referring, presumably, to the UK),

> [w]e made a democratic decision to provide collective cover: the costs we incur as a result are down to us . . . [Moreover] the legislation does not exempt people who are prepared to eliminate extra costs to others by taking out private insurance, or simply by waiving their right to be treated in case of accident.

Skorupski's argument seems to suggest that whenever a society democratically introduces a compulsory public healthcare system, citizens (and their representatives) are (or, at least, should be) aware of the fact that many (probably most) people do engage in activities that may involve risks and potentially lead to greater healthcare costs for the public. Those people might be asked from the beginning to contribute a larger than average share of the overall costs of the system, but if they are not (as happens in most cases), then they cannot subsequently be asked to pay that additional price.

Since collective healthcare cover, where it exists, is normally established democratically, one might argue that citizens should also have the right to democratically remove it or renegotiate it (and many countries indeed regularly reform their healthcare systems). However, as long as there is democratic consensus on compulsory collective cover without exceptions, it seems unfair to 'punish' risk-takers, e.g. through financial penalties.

Finally, even if it was ascertained that some eaters' dietary patterns represent a net cost for society, that this constitutes a harm to society, and that these eaters therefore ought to bear the costs of their 'irresponsible' choices, this would justify only tailored penalties but not over-inclusive measures, such as sugary drink taxes, which would inevitably also penalize individuals whose conduct does not harm others in any way. As Riley (1998, p. 200) suggests, 'self-financing private-sector insurance schemes could in principle be designed so that different classes of consumers would pay different premiums according to the risks which they, respectively, choose to bear'. This solution would be similar to the one we suggested earlier with regard to negligent individuals who have voluntarily undertaken obligations towards their family or creditors. In this case, it would extend to those individuals who, while not having undertaken any voluntary obligations towards others, have made dietary choices that have harmful financial repercussions on the public healthcare system (assuming, as we said earlier, that Mill's conception of harm can be stretched to such an extent).

Private insurance schemes such as those proposed by Riley are more consistent with Mill's account than uniform compulsory public healthcare, and are, e.g., already in place in the US, where most individuals receive private insurance offered by their employers through group coverage schemes. Interestingly, empirical research has shown that even though in the US the insurance premiums of employees who are obese and who are under group coverage are not normally increased to reflect the greater healthcare costs often associated with obesity, 'obese workers with employer-sponsored health insurance pay for their higher expected medical expenditures through lower cash wages' (Bhattacharya and Bundorf 2009, p. 657; see also Cawley 2004).[9] Further research may show in the future that similar wage penalties are also informally applied to other categories of employees who present other diet-related conditions which lead to greater healthcare costs. Conversely, some US companies have begun to reward their non-overweight employees with lower health insurance premiums (e.g. see Anonymous 2012c). These kinds of penalties and rewards, if applied with the aim of offsetting greater healthcare costs due to 'irresponsible' eating, seem to be legitimate from a Millian perspective: they target those whose dietary patterns cause increased healthcare costs but, unlike indiscriminate measures such as sugary drink taxes, they

---

[9] While the authors of this research acknowledge that this may be partly due to informal discrimination against obese workers, they also point out that it is mostly female workers who are affected by these wage differences. Their explanation is that '[t]he difference in the average health expenditures between the obese and the non-obese is larger for adult women than for adult men. Obese women spent $1457 more per year on healthcare than did non-obese women; the analogous difference for men is $405' (Bhattacharya and Bundorf 2009, p. 655). In other words, their explanation is that female workers who are obese receive lower wages because they impose higher costs than their male counterparts on group coverage, rather than due to gender discrimination. However, this conclusion seems problematic, and indeed the authors themselves do not entirely rule out discrimination as a potential factor (p. 655). Our main point is that if and when other factors like discrimination can be ruled out, lower cash wages for obese workers with employer-sponsored health insurance may be consistent with a Millian approach.

do not affect those individuals whose dietary patterns (e.g. eating unhealthy foods in moderation) do not 'harm' society through increased healthcare costs. Of course, this assumes (a big assumption) that overweight is a suitable proxy for increased healthcare costs associated with dietary patterns; i.e. this assumes that by targeting those who are overweight (rather than those who have a kind of dietary pattern known to be associated with diet-related illness and increased healthcare costs) the insurance companies are accurately targeting those whose dietary patterns cause increased healthcare costs. Also, once again, this conclusion presupposes the view that the extra healthcare costs for society caused by people with unhealthy dietary patterns do indeed *harm* society—a view which, we explained earlier, some may challenge.

3.6. Taxing unhealthy foods: Mill and 'secondary paternalism'

Thus far we have argued that Mill's theory would warrant a number of measures targeting unhealthy eaters whose conduct causes some kind of harm to others. Mill's arguments, therefore, seem to justify only tailored measures that penalize people with unhealthy dietary patterns, while ruling out indiscriminate measures like fast food or sugary drink taxes. Consumption of unhealthy foods is not intrinsically associated with harmful other-regarding conduct. It seems that it would therefore be unjust, from a Millian perspective, to prohibit the consumption of unhealthy foods or render it more difficult for everyone, e.g. by imposing a tax upon them. This would unwarrantedly penalize all those individuals whose consumption of unhealthy foods does not prevent them from fulfilling their obligations (towards their family, employer, creditors, etc.) and does not render them a burden for the public healthcare system. As Riley (1998, p. 101) highlights,

> the extravagant man who nevertheless is able to pay his debts, the public servant who is drunk only while off duty and the cocaine addict who is as kind and helpful to others as they may reasonably expect under prevailing social conventions, should remain perfectly free from legal or social penalties.

Yet, quite surprisingly, Mill ([1859] 2006, p. 113) also provides a justification for taxing unhealthy foods. Indeed in one of his few remarks on alcohol, he argues the following:

To tax stimulants for the sole purpose of making them more difficult to be obtained, is a measure differing only in degree from their entire prohibition; and would be justifiable only if that were justifiable. Every increase of cost is a prohibition, to those whose means do not come up to the augmented price; and to those who do, it is a penalty laid on them for gratifying a particular taste.

However, he then also adds

that taxation for fiscal purposes is absolutely inevitable; that in most countries it is necessary that a considerable part of that taxation should be indirect;[10] that the State, therefore, cannot help imposing penalties, which to some persons may be prohibitory, on the use of some articles of consumption. It is hence the duty of the State to consider, in the imposition of taxes, what commodities the consumers can best spare; and à fortiori, to select in preference those of which it deems the use, beyond a very moderate quantity, to be positively injurious. Taxation, therefore, of stimulants, up to the point which produces the largest amount of revenue (supposing that the State needs all the revenue which it yields) is not only admissible, but to be approved of. (p. 114)

Here Mill seems to have been partly inspired by Adam Smith's ([1776] 1904, V.3.76) view that '[s]ugar, rum, and tobacco are commodities which are nowhere necessaries of life, which are become objects of almost universal consumption, and which are therefore extremely proper subjects of taxation.' Smith's conclusion may be one of the first examples of a 'sugar tax' proposal. Yet there is a crucial difference between Smith's and Mill's arguments. While Smith highlights the *superfluous* nature of the goods he believes should be taxed, Mill explicitly emphasizes that the state has a duty (if and when indirect taxation is required) to impose indirect taxation upon those goods whose excessive consumption may cause *self-regarding harm*. Mill's conclusion therefore justifies what we would like to call 'secondary paternalism'. The criterion for indirect taxation advocated by Mill does not indicate that paternalistic interventions should be the primary goal of the state. However, it

---

[10] According to Mill [1848] (1965b, p. 825) '[t]axes are either direct or indirect. A direct tax is one which is demanded from the very persons who, it is intended or desired, should pay it. Indirect taxes are those which are demanded from one person in the expectation and intention that he shall indemnify himself at the expense of another: such as the excise or customs'.

does suggest that appealing to paternalistic reasons is permissible, and in fact required, when deciding to which goods indirect taxes should be applied (if indirect taxation is required at all).

It is true that Mill's ([1859] 2006, p. 114) qualification ('supposing that the State needs all the revenue which it yields') potentially limits the scope of indirect taxation. If the state had other ways of raising revenue (e.g. through direct taxation), then it should not violate the freedom of buyers by imposing these sales taxes upon them. Even so, Mill could have quite easily proposed a different criterion for deciding which goods should be taxed, *if* the state definitely needed to raise additional revenue through indirect taxation. For example, he could have fully embraced Smith's distinction between essential and superfluous goods, and argued that only the latter should be taxed, regardless of whether they are 'positively injurious' (p. 114) when consumed beyond a very small amount. By choosing the 'positively injurious' criterion, which also applies to unhealthy foods, Mill therefore implicitly justifies the permissibility of taxes on foods that are 'positively injurious' (e.g. a sugary drink tax) and of all analogous forms of indirect taxation which also penalize and restrict the freedom of 'responsible' eaters.

There is, however, a further point to be observed. One of the main problems raised by sugary drink taxes and, more generally, by any taxes on food, is that they tend to be especially regressive. Even though Mill does not address this issue in *On Liberty*, he does consider it in the *Principles of Political Economy*. He argues there that '[t]ea, coffee, sugar, tobacco, fermented drinks, can hardly be so taxed that the poor shall not bear more than their due share of the burthen' (Mill [1848] 1965b, p. 870). Unhealthy foods can easily be added to this list. Mill therefore suggests that the regressive nature of this kind of indirect taxation could be partly offset 'by making the duty on the superior qualities, which are used by the richer consumers, much higher in proportion to the value' (p. 870). This might entail, we suppose, applying a higher duty on whisky than on lager, on luxury chocolate than on cheap chocolate bars, on high-quality red meat than on fast foods, etc.

Mill ([1848] 1965b, p. 871), however, acknowledges that this solution would often be impractical and that the easier option of applying the same duty on all products, regardless of their quality, entails 'a flagrant injustice to the poorer class of contributors, unless compensated by the existence of other taxes from which, as from the present income tax, they are altogether exempt'. Mill's account therefore implies not that indirect taxes should be avoided altogether but that they should be as progressive as possible, or at least accompanied by a regime of direct taxation aimed at offsetting their regressive features. Mill's concern for lower income people, therefore, does not constitute a decisive obstacle to the indirect taxation of unhealthy foods. It only implies that such taxes should be levied as fairly as possible. This leaves Mill's 'secondary paternalism' unaltered.

3.7. Millian liberalism, food advertising, and food labelling

We finally consider the implications of Mill's perfectionist liberalism for the regulation of food advertising and food labelling. Mill's position regarding advertising is slightly ambiguous. On the one hand, he argues that individuals should be allowed to advise each other to do the things they are allowed to do (i.e. within the limits imposed by the harm principle) (Mill [1859] 2006, p. 111). On the other hand, however, he argues that '[t]he question is doubtful, only when the instigator derives a personal benefit from his advice; when he makes it his occupation, for subsistence or pecuniary gain, to promote what society and the State consider to be an evil' (p. 111). Buyers, that is, should be able to make their purchases 'as free as possible from the arts of persons who stimulate their inclinations for interested purposes of their own' (p. 112). In the case of alcohol, e.g. even though sales restrictions should not be implemented, as that would also unduly restrict the freedom of buyers, Mill argues that '[t]he interests ... of [strong drink] dealers in promoting intemperance is a real evil, and justifies the State in imposing restrictions and requiring guarantees which, but for that justification, would be infringements of legitimate liberty' (p. 113). This suggests that Mill would have probably justified imposing restrictions upon the advertising of unhealthy foods, when such restrictions aim to constrain the producers' goal to promote the excessive consumption of those foods.

This is especially relevant to the issue of food advertisements directed at children, for two main reasons. First, as we observed earlier, it should be noted that the harm principle, for Mill ([1859] 2006, p. 16), does not apply to 'children, or . . . young persons below the age which the law may fix as that of manhood or womanhood'. As children (unlike adults) should not be free, for Mill, to engage in behaviour that concerns only themselves and their interests, similarly they should not be free 'to exchange opinions, and give and receive suggestions' (p. 111) concerning that behaviour. Second, it is well known that '[c]orporations . . . have a vested interest in targeting younger and younger consumers and invest billions both in advertising and product placement' (Merry 2012, p. 2). The state may therefore legitimately impose restrictions upon adverts for sugary cereals, sugary drinks, and other un-healthy foods that target children and young people. This is the case, e.g. in the UK where 'a ban on advertising "junk" foods before, during and after educational TV programmes aimed at children' (Wickins-Drazilova and Williams 2011, p. 15) has already been implemented. Such measures may contribute to changing the 'obesogenic environment' (Voigt 2012, p. 2) which strongly conditions parents' ability to make dietary choices on behalf of their children (Merry 2012, p. 5). However, these restrictions also have limits. As Wickins-Drazilova and Williams (2011, p. 16) highlight, the omnipresent character of marketing implies that in spite of any restrictions, children are still likely to be exposed to some form of advertising, 'from supermarkets through bill-boards to the internet and disguised advertising in the form of "product placement" in many film and television shows' (see also Voigt et al. 2014, pp. 154–72).

One might suggest, of course, that these marketing tools should be re-stricted too. However, we should remember, as we noted earlier, that the harm principle is for Mill ([1859] 2006, p. 18) a necessary but not sufficient condition for interfering with the liberty of others, and that 'the attempt to exercise control [i.e. in this case, to regulate extensively corporations' mar-keting strategies] would [probably, for Mill] produce other evils, greater than those which it would prevent'. It might significantly reduce, e.g., the freedom of adult consumers to be informed about different products they may wish to purchase.[11] In summary, while Mill would have certainly endorsed some restrictions, he probably would not have justified systematic state control over food advertising.

More complex, however, are the implications of Mill's theory for leg-islation concerning food labels. Consider, e.g., nutrition facts labels, men-tioned in Chapter 1. Such labels are now compulsory for all packaged food products in several countries, and their purpose is to ensure that consumers are fully informed about the nutritional value of the foods they eat. This is

---

[11] An alternative solution might therefore be for the state to 'be more concerned with developing children's ability to respond to advertising intelligently, than with the (probably vain) attempt to pre-vent their being exposed to it' (Wickins-Drazilova and Williams 2011, p. 16).

apparently in line with Mill's account. The passage in *On Liberty* that is most closely related to nutrition facts labels is Mill's ([1859] 2006, p. 109) view that, when dealing with the sale of poisons, '[s]uch a precaution ... as that of labelling the drug with some word expressive of its dangerous character, may be enforced without violation of liberty; the buyer cannot wish not to know that the thing he possesses has poisonous qualities'. Similarly, nutrition facts labels are necessary to ensure that consumers are fully aware of the implications of their actions and voluntarily choose to perform them (even if these actions are 'bad' or dangerous for them). From a Millian perspective, then, consumers can legitimately be warned about the nutritional value of the foods they choose to eat.

Yet one might suggest that the analogy between unhealthy food and poison is imperfect because many people in fact do wish to ignore the long-term effects of the foods they eat (e.g. Bonotti 2014; Loi 2014). More precisely, one could argue that many people do not wish *to be reminded of* those effects. Being constantly warned about the high saturated fat or high sugar contents of one's favourite meals may seriously undermine one's enjoyment of those foods. If that is the case, one might argue, food labelling is paternalistic, at least towards those people who wish to remain ignorant or not to be reminded about the long-term effects of their food. This remark clearly relies on an empirical assumption which may be difficult to prove or disprove. One would need to carry out surveys, collect data, etc., in order to establish what people's attitude to their food consumption actually is and what they wish or do not wish to know about its effects. On these grounds, however, one might also contest Mill's ([1859] 2006, p.109) own assumption that the purchaser 'cannot wish not to know' the poisonous nature of the substance they buy.

Similarly, Mill ([1859] 2006, p. 109) also argues that

> [i]f either a public officer or any one else saw a person attempting to cross a bridge which had been ascertained to be unsafe, and there were no time to warn him of his danger, they might seize him and turn him back, without any real infringement of his liberty; for liberty consists in doing what one desires, and he does not desire to fall into the river.

But the empirical assumption behind these examples, one might argue, is flawed because Mill does not take into account those cases in which a person willingly chooses to adopt a risky behaviour such as walking across an unsafe bridge or using poisonous substances while also willingly choosing to remain ignorant of the exact degree and kind of risk involved.

However, we may not need to rest our conclusions about these cases on empirical assumptions about how many people wish to remain ignorant about the dangers they face. There are other variables at stake in the three examples. In the bridge example, the danger faced by the agent is both certain (the bridge 'had been ascertained to be unsafe') (Mill [1859] 2006, p. 109) and imminent (there is 'no time to warn him of his danger') (p. 109). For Mill, this justifies 'soft paternalism' (Feinberg 1986), i.e. stopping that person in order to warn them and ensure that their action is voluntary and well informed. Once we have ensured that the person is fully aware of the situation, then we should leave them free, from Mill's point of view, to cross the bridge and fall into the river if they wish so. Mill's ([1859] 2006, p. 109) statement that the person 'does not desire to fall into the river' is perhaps unfortunate in its 'absolute' tone, but we believe it should be interpreted in the following way: most people most of the time do not wish to fall into rivers, and even if a minority of them does, we have a right to temporarily interfere with a person's freedom in order to ascertain whether she belongs to that minority and is aware of the consequences of her actions. Some individuals may then decide to cross the bridge, and we should leave them free to do so.

The poisons example presents a different scenario. Here the danger is not imminent (i.e. the person is not about to drink the poison, only to purchase it), and it is not certain (i.e. the person may use the poison for non-dangerous goals, e.g. 'to help protect the plants in his garden from insects' (Riley 1998, p. 121)). In such cases, Mill ([1859] 2006, p. 109) argues, 'no one but the person himself can judge of the sufficiency of the motive which may prompt him to incur the risk: in this case, therefore, (unless he is a child, or delirious, or in some state of excitement or absorption incompatible with the full use of the reflecting faculty) he ought . . . to be only warned of the danger; not forcibly prevented from exposing himself to it'. Therefore, we cannot forbid the sale of the product or even 'require in all cases the certificate of a medical practitioner' (p. 109) but only warn them about the product's dangerous nature through labelling.

Once again, we believe that Mill's ([1859] 2006, p. 109) strong statement that 'the buyer cannot wish not to know that the thing he possesses has poisonous qualities' should be interpreted in the following way: most people most of the time wish to be informed about the poisonous effects of the goods they purchase, and even if a minority of them does not, we have a right to temporarily interfere (through labelling) with a person's freedom in order to ascertain whether she belongs to that minority and is aware of the consequences of her actions. Once we have applied the warning label on the poison package we should leave buyers free to purchase the poison and use it for self-harming actions. However, given the potential other-regarding harm that may derive from the use of the poison (e.g. the buyer may use it to kill someone else), Mill also recommends that '[t]he seller . . . might be required to enter in a register the exact time of the transaction, the name and address of the buyer, the precise quality and quantity sold; to ask the purpose for which it was wanted, and record the answer he received' (p. 110).

The case of food labelling is different from the previous cases only in degree. The danger associated with eating unhealthy food is much less certain and imminent than that incurred by crossing an unsafe bridge or by using a poisonous substance unaware of its effects (e.g. see Conly 2013a, pp. 154, 167). Accordingly, the interference upon the agent's action should be milder, and this is what nutrition facts labels aim to ensure. This, however, requires a clarification. The labelling of poisons recommended by Mill ([1859] 2006, p. 109), we have seen, should include 'some word expressive of its dangerous character'. This is because the poison is certainly and immediately dangerous *if* drunk or ingested. To be sure, this is also the case of certain foods, not necessarily unhealthy ones. There seem to be good reasons, e.g., for providing clear and explicit labels which state whether a food product contains nuts or other potentially allergenic ingredients.

Yet, apart from these cases, which closely resemble Mill's example of poisons and thus warrant visible and explicit food labels, most foods (including unhealthy ones) are generally unlikely to cause immediate and certain dangers to one's health. From a Millian perspective, therefore, it seems that nutrition facts labels should be 'milder' than poison labels. They should provide only objective information about the nutrients contained in the foods one purchases rather than explicit warnings (analogous to the message 'Smoking kills' found on cigarette packets) such as 'This food will kill you in the long term', 'If you eat too much of this food you are likely to die of a heart attack/of cancer', or even graphic pictures of the health conditions that eating certain foods could potentially cause (e.g. Stephens 2014). The use of milder labels with objective nutrition information would still allow those consumers who want to find out whether the nutritional contents of their foods are good or bad for their health to investigate what information the nutrition facts labels contain and what this entails. However, it would also avoid interfering with the freedom of those who want to remain ignorant or wish not to be reminded about the health effects of their foods, and who may consider overly explicit and/or graphic nutrition labels paternalistic.

This conclusion, however, may be too rushed. Even though it may be true that many individuals would rather remain ignorant (or not be reminded) about the effects of the unhealthy foods they eat, it is not entirely clear whether a Millian state should accommodate their demands, i.e. by forbidding the provision of explicit or even graphic warning labels on foods. Indeed Mill ([1859] 2006, p. 86) argues that '[h]uman beings owe to each other help to distinguish the better from the worse, and encouragement to choose the former and avoid the latter'. According to Skorupski (1999, p. 222), this implies that 'human beings . . . have a moral obligation [e.g. a duty to educate each other]: something which . . . society can enforce'. Food labels, even of the more explicit and graphic kinds, may therefore be seen as a means of persuasion that society and the state can legitimately use in order to persuade people not to consume certain foods. In other words, while the Millian state ought to be 'permissively neutral' (Skorupski 1999, p. 223), i.e. it should not prevent individuals from pursuing their preferred conceptions of the good, or impose upon them any such conception(s), it need not embrace 'persuasive neutrality' (p. 223). The latter consists of 'refrain[ing] from taking any part in the discussion or advancement of ethical ideals, whether as the proponent of some particular ideals or as the patron of some such proponents' (p. 223). If the Millian state, therefore, believes that it is better for individuals to lead a healthy lifestyle (e.g. because by being healthy and living longer they have a greater chance to develop their individual autonomy and cultivate an independent character[12]), then it may legitimately persuade them to do so, even if some (or many) of them would rather not listen to its advice. It is true that such persuasive measures may reduce the enjoyment of those eaters who would rather remain ignorant about the unhealthiness of their foods. Yet it is also true that accommodating these eaters' preferences may seriously undermine the effectiveness of food labels, as most consumers (who would rather know what is in their foods) may ignore 'milder' nutrition facts labels and be persuaded only by more explicit and graphic ones.

---

[12] The emphasis on individual autonomy and on the cultivation of an independent character, some might argue, already presupposes a perfectionist view, thus reducing the scope of Mill's 'permissive neutrality' (Skorupski 1999, p. 223). We set this issue aside here.

One might also add that sometimes people rank the potential evil consequences of their choices irrationally (Gert and Culver 1979, pp. 205–7), and that perhaps those who would prefer not to be informed about the unhealthy effects of their foods are acting irrationally. Sarah Conly, e.g., takes up the issue of the rationality of food choices. She points out that

> if we knew we were going to follow our burger and fries with an immediate heart attack . . . none of us would eat it, no matter how strong our cravings, just as we won't drink antifreeze, no matter how thirsty. When this meal is only one out of a very long series, though, no one of which strikes the fatal blow, we find it easier to dismiss. (Conly 2013a, p. 167)

The risk associated with eating unhealthy foods is therefore more incremental than the risk associated, say, with crossing an unsafe bridge, as in Mill's example. Moreover, Conly's conclusion assumes that virtually no person wishes to die of heart attack or similar health conditions. If Conly is right, then her argument may justify not only explicit food labels but also more coercive healthy eating efforts. Indeed, according to her, Mill overestimates people's ability to think rationally (p. 55). Due to people's poor reasoning, she claims, food labelling is often ineffective in persuading eaters to adopt healthier dietary habits. She therefore concludes that more coercive paternalistic measures, such as reducing food portions in restaurants, would be both justified and more effective in promoting healthier eating amongst the population than less coercive measures such as food labelling (pp. 167–69).

In response, one might argue that it is rational—or at least not too irrational (or uncommon)—to be willing to accept a shorter life in order to be able to enjoy the unhealthy (and tasty) food one likes (Finkelstein and Zuckerman 2008, pp. 82–91). Conly (2013a, p. 157) herself highlights how soda consumption restrictions (such as the policy of excluding sugary drinks from food assistance programmes, which many US states have proposed) can cause a real 'loss of enjoyment' amongst soda drinkers, and she thinks that this kind of psychological cost should be taken into account when assessing the appropriateness of paternalistic policies. But even granting that unhealthy dietary patterns *are* irrational, as Conly thinks they generally are, this does not mean that Mill would have supported coercive measures to prevent consumption of unhealthy foods, in addition to explicit food labels. Since Mill argues that we should leave people free to commit suicide by crossing unsafe bridges once informed, however irrational that might be (e.g. see Riley 1998, p. 121), he would have also presumably argued that we should leave people free to incur long-term diet-related health risks if they wish so, once they have been informed about the risks associated with their unhealthy dietary patterns through explicit food labels.

An additional Millian argument in support of explicit food labels can be built on Powers et al.'s (2012) suggestion that Mill's theory would justify the regulation of the marketplace for the sake of public health. Powers et al. argue that while Mill thought that there *is* a conclusive presumption in favour of some liberties—such as liberty of expression—there is not 'a blanket presumption in favor of liberty in all matters of state action for the sake of the public's health' (p. 7). On their view, Mill was centrally concerned with individual self-determination—i.e. individuals developing their capacities to determine their own destinies, and developing and executing a plan of life. Self-determination in this sense requires certain liberties—'liberties that protect the kinds of choices that structure the contours of one's life in their most fundamentally defining ways' (p. 9)—but does *not* require unrestricted liberty in the marketplace. Protecting the liberties important to Mill is compatible with regulating the marketplace for the sake of public health, since 'the choices routinely implicated in public welfare regulation are without deep moral significance for the broad contours of a life that qualifies as substantially self-determining' (p. 10).

Powers et al.'s (2012) more nuanced understanding of Mill's theory therefore seems to offer an additional Millian argument in favour of explicit food labels. However, we should be careful in overestimating the implications of their conclusion. While some forms of public health regulation, such as food labelling, might be considered to have little 'deep moral significance' for individuals' self-development, since they do not ultimately undermine people's ability to pursue their chosen life plans, more coercive healthy eating efforts could infringe on such ability. As we observed in Chapter 1, food and eating habits, including unhealthy ones, *are* central to many people's life plans, and therefore *are* related to the 'kinds of choices that structure the contours of one's life in their most fundamentally defining ways' (p. 9). This is, we believe, one of the aspects that have been mostly overlooked in the current normative debates on healthy eating policy.

In sum, the analysis conducted in this chapter suggests that Mill would have accepted warning and persuasive healthy eating measures (e.g. food labels, including explicit and graphic ones), but not coercive measures such as limiting food portion sizes or the banning of certain foods. This does not mean, though, that Mill would not have accepted paternalistic healthy eating interventions *tout court*. As we argued earlier, the limited paternalism that he endorses in relation to indirect taxation—what we labelled 'secondary paternalism'—does support some such measures. However, the overall analysis conducted in this chapter suggests that his endorsement of 'secondary paternalism' is clearly at odds with the rest of his theory of liberty, and should be seen more as an unfortunate inconsistency than as a defining feature of that theory, and of its implications for healthy eating policy.

A primary objection to Mill's liberal approach, we pointed out, is that it overestimates the extent to which people can control their eating habits, and neglects the social, psychological, physiological, and environmental influences on eating behaviour. This significantly reduces the usefulness of a liberty-centred theory for critically assessing healthy eating efforts. In the next chapter, we will show how this flaw also affects contemporary anti-paternalism accounts, thus pointing towards the need for a perspective shift in the analysis of healthy eating efforts.

4

Healthy Eating Efforts and Paternalism

4.1. Introduction

This chapter introduces and critically discusses debates about paternalism and healthy eating efforts, which have been prominent in bioethics and political philosophy. 'Healthy eating efforts' are defined broadly in this book to include a range of efforts by the state (and other actors) to shift dietary patterns in healthier directions. Some efforts focus on changing the mix of foods in our daily food environments, such as incentivizing stores to stock a healthier mix of foods, changing the mix of foods in vending machines in schools and workplaces, or limiting the density of fast-food restaurants. Others concentrate on food marketing, trying to limit food advertising towards children or the kinds of foods that can be marketed; to stop companies from targeting some groups with heavier marketing (e.g. African Americans); or to counteract food marketing with clear and compelling nutrition labels and warnings. Another category of efforts aims to change which products are brought to market or the price of those products, such as bans on trans fat in packaged food and restaurant food, and taxes on sugary drinks. Other efforts focus on changing how people interact with their food environments, such as nutrition education, counselling, or other individual-focused interventions. Finally, some healthy eating efforts focus on the food supply chain (e.g. calls to increase fruit and vegetable production) or target broader social and economic factors that influence health (e.g. increasing access to healthcare, improving public transportation, and reducing poverty); however, we are not much concerned here with these latter two kinds of efforts.

As we showed in Chapter 1, some healthy eating efforts raise 'nanny state' complaints, as in the case of the failed NYC soda ban in 2020. We also saw that defenders of healthy eating efforts sometimes respond to charges of 'nannying' by arguing that such efforts do not patronizingly protect consumers from themselves but rather from a misleading, deceiving, manipulating food industry, or that charges of 'nannying' are the result of the food

Healthy Eating Policy and Political Philosophy. Anne Barnhill and Matteo Bonotti, Oxford University Press. © Oxford University Press 2022. DOI: 10.1093/oso/9780190937881.003.0005

industry working behind the scenes to shape public opinion. But charges of nannying and related criticisms reflect long-standing ethical objections to government paternalism, and these objections deserve serious consideration.

This chapter examines two objections to government paternalism in some detail: Jonathan Quong's objection that it fails to treat people as 'free and equal', and the objection that it is perfectionist, i.e. that it advances a controversial conception of the good (see Chapter 2). The chapter considers how those objections apply to healthy eating efforts, and responds to those objections.

4.2. What is paternalism?

'Paternalism' is defined in multiple, distinct ways in the literature. One understanding of paternalism characterizes it as 'the interference with a person's liberty of action justified by reasons referring exclusively to the welfare, good, happiness, needs, interests or values of the person being coerced' (Quong 2011, pp. 74–75, quoting Dworkin 1972). Following Quong, we call this paternalism in the 'liberty-limiting' sense. This definition has influenced (explicitly or implicitly) the debate on public health paternalism both in public life and in the scholarly literature, including the debate on healthy eating efforts. However, as Quong points out, paternalism so defined does not capture those instances when we seem to be acting paternalistically without limiting another person's freedom. For instance, Quong provides the example of someone offering to take her boyfriend out to his favourite restaurant if he spends the afternoon working on the paper that he should be working on, because she does not believe he will do it otherwise. This action, in Quong's view (and we agree with him) is paternalistic even though it is not liberty-limiting.

Quong (2011, p. 80) therefore defines paternalism

as any act where:
1. Agent A attempts to improve the welfare, good, happiness, needs, interests, or values of agent B with regard to a particular decision or situation that B faces.
2. A's act is motivated by a negative judgment about B's ability (assuming B has the relevant information) to make the right decision or manage the

particular situation in a way that will effectively advance B's welfare, good, happiness, needs, interests, or values.

According to Quong (2011, p. 81), this definition captures 'the essence of what we mean when we use the term. It captures our sense that to treat someone paternalistically is to treat that person like a child in the specific sense of acting in that person's best interests because you believe, in this situation, the person lacks the ability to do so himself or herself'. In other words, acting paternalistically involves 'holding a negative judgment about the paternalizee's capacity to effectively advance his or her own interests' (p. 83). The abilities that Quong considers relevant to this judgemental definition are 'practical reasoning, willpower, and emotion management' (p. 81).

We prefer Quong's definition of paternalism to the liberty-limiting one because many of the efforts we are concerned with—and which have provoked the charge of 'nannying'—are not liberty-limiting. Thus Quong's definition seems to better capture those instances of concern. Some healthy eating efforts (e.g. food bans, sugary drink taxes, or other taxes) reduce in different ways people's liberty, but others (e.g. incentives/disincentives, information/education, nudges) do not, even though they would be considered by many to also be paternalistic. Indeed, the charge of 'nannying', which reflects the concern that policies treat the public as if they were children and paternalize them, is applied to many healthy eating efforts, not just those that limit liberty.

4.3. Objections to paternalism

In the philosophical literature and in the bioethics literature, a number of objections are lodged to government paternalism.

One objection is that people know best what will advance their own interests; thus, paternalistic action by the government that interferes with people's actions is not likely to be an improvement on letting people alone to make decisions for themselves (e.g. Mill [1859] 2006). Some defenders of paternalism respond by arguing that there is ample evidence that people regularly act in ways that undermine their own ends and that shaping people's actions (through coercion or through nudges) can help them better achieve their own ends or goals (Conly 2013a; Sunstein 2014).

A second kind of objection is that paternalism is insulting or disrespectful or fails to treat the paternalized person as an equal (for discussion and critique of this class of objections, see Conly 2013a and Hanna 2018). Sarah Conly (2013b, pp. 241–42) articulates a version of this objection:

> interfering with people's actions make[s] the morally suspect claim that people are fundamentally unequal in their abilities. It has been said of paternalism that it involves an unacceptable substitution of judgment, where one person (or set of persons) substitutes his (their) superior judgment for the inferior judgment shown by the person who will otherwise take the dangerous action.

Conly responds to this objection by arguing that while 'paternalism involves a substitution of judgment about means to ends . . . in these circumstances such a substitution does not suggest any kind of inequality between persons' (p. 241). Paternalism could be rooted in the view that we all, equally, experience certain failures of reasoning and self-governance, and we all need help (i.e. paternalistic policies) to mitigate this.

A related objection is that 'paternalism promotes inequality between people, and that coercive paternalism, in particular, actually establishes structures that enforce inequality' (Conly 2013b, p. 242). In other words, government paternalism creates a class of government paternalizers with power over everyone else. A response to this objection is that we need not designate some people as decision-makers who tell the rest of us what to do, willy-nilly. Instead, we should have laws and policies preventing us from doing self-destructive things (e.g. laws mandating banning cigarettes, or mandating that people wear seat belts) (Conly 2013b).

This brings us to another objection to government paternalism: those who design paternalistic policy—who are only human, after all—will have the same failures of reasoning and decision-making as the people whom they are designing policy for (Waldron 2014). Therefore, we should not expect paternalistic policy to be much of an improvement over leaving people to their own devices. This objection, however, seems to confuse the failures of reasoning and decision-making that people experience situationally in their everyday lives (e.g. people over-consume sugary foods in irrational ways in contemporary food environments, or they irrationally choose the French fries rather than the salad in the cafeteria line) with the rather distinct kinds of failures of reasoning and decision-making that would be relevant to designing sound policy (e.g. failures of statistical reasoning), which could be addressed through sound policymaking processes.

There are also autonomy-based objections to government paternalism. One such objection is that government paternalism can undermine the individual's development and exercise of autonomy and is unjustifiable for this reason. That is, a person developing and exercising individual autonomy is so important that the government should not interfere with her autonomous actions, even to prevent the person from harming herself (see Arneson 1980; Dworkin 1972; Feinberg 1986; Kleinig 1984; VanDeVeer 1986). A general response to autonomy-based objections is that these objections may be rooted in substantive views about the importance of autonomy and its place in a good life—views that may not be widely shared in pluralistic societies. For example, the view that a person developing and exercising individual autonomy is more important than that person being protected from harm is a substantive conception of the good life, and one that many people would reject. When government paternalism is rejected on the basis of this kind of substantive conception of the good life, this arguably fails from the perspective of public reason. Recall, from Chapter 2, that 'public reason' is the view that state laws and policies can be implemented only if they are justified on the basis of reasons that are public, i.e. reasons that all citizens can accept at some level of idealization despite their different conceptions of the good. (In Chapters 5–7 we will provide a more detailed discussion of public reason and the justification for healthy eating efforts.)

Indeed Rawls (2005a) argues more than once that Millian and Kantian conceptions of autonomy, which are centred around the reflective and critical use of our deliberative faculties, are controversial. Like religious doctrines, these controversial views cannot offer public reasons for government policy. Similarly, writing in the context of debates on freedom of expression, Joshua Cohen (1993, p. 222) argues:

> [The view that] expression always trumps other values because of its connection with autonomy . . . suggests that a commitment to freedom of expression turns on embracing the supreme value of autonomy. But this threatens to turn freedom of expression into a sectarian political position. Is a strong commitment to expressive liberties really available only to those who endorse the idea that autonomy is the fundamental human good—an idea about which there is much reasonable controversy? I am not doubting

that such a strong commitment is available to those whose ethical views are of this kind, but I reject the claim that such views are really necessary.

This does not mean, of course, that the value of autonomy should play no role in the public justification of state policies, including healthy eating efforts. While rejecting comprehensive conceptions of autonomy, for example, Rawls (2005a, p. 19) argues that one of our key moral powers 'is the capacity to form, to revise and rationally to pursue a conception of one's rational advantage or good'. This can be understood as a 'milder', and therefore less controversial, conception of individual autonomy than those endorsed by Mill and Kant. To say that paternalism violates our ability to exercise milder autonomy is certainly a relevant consideration in public reasoning. Yet to claim that this should be an *overriding* consideration, as many anti-paternalists might seem to argue, involves a failure of public reason. As we will argue in later chapters, public reasoning involves the balancing of different political values, and this entails that sometimes we can partly hinder the realization of some of these values to the benefit of others.

An additional objection to paternalism, we have already mentioned, is provided by Quong. This is the view that paternalism fails to treat people as free and equal (in a Rawlsian sense); we discuss this in section 4.4. A further objection to paternalistic public health efforts, which we consider in section 4.6, is that they are perfectionist in a sense.

4.4. Quong's objection to paternalism in the 'judgemental' sense

According to Quong (2011, p. 74), paternalism (in the judgemental sense) is presumptively wrong 'because of the way it denies someone's status as a free and equal citizen'. Recall that paternalism, as we follow Quong in defining it, rests on a negative judgement about B's ability to make the right decision or manage the particular situation in a way that will effectively advance B's welfare, good, happiness, needs, interests, or values (and, we would add, a negative judgement about B's ability to make decisions or manage situations in ways that enact and cohere with B's life plan and conception of the good). When governments are motivated by such judgements, Quong argues, they fail to treat citizens as if they have the capacity for a conception of the good, which is 'the capacity to form, to revise, and rationally to pursue a conception of one's rational advantage or good' (pp. 100–101). Quong is here adopting a requirement highlighted by Rawls, 'to act in accordance with principles that are consistent with, and give expression to, this conception of citizens as free and equal' (Quong 2011, p. 101). Paternalism does not seem to do this, according to Quong, because 'it treats citizens as if they cannot make effective decisions about their own good, and thereby diminishes the moral status accorded to citizens' (p. 103). Let's dig into Quong's objection to paternalistic policies, evaluate it, and consider its application to healthy eating efforts.

Assessing Quong's objection will involve considering whether (and which) healthy eating efforts are paternalistic in Quong's sense: first, whether (and which of) these efforts aim to improve people's welfare, and second, whether (and which of) these efforts are based on a negative judgement about people's ability to make the right decisions or advance their own welfare. After considering whether (and which) healthy eating efforts are paternalistic in Quong's sense, we will then consider whether this does actually run afoul, in a meaningful way, of the Rawlsian requirement that governments treat members of the public as if they have 'the capacity to form, to revise, and rationally to pursue a conception of one's rational advantage or good' (Quong 2011, pp. 100–101).

First, which healthy eating efforts aim to improve people's welfare? This is a surprisingly complicated question. Some healthy eating efforts have multiple immediate aims, including the aim of improving the targeted population's health but also other aims. For example, some sugary drink taxes proposed or implemented in US cities and states plausibly aim to improve the health of the population subjected to the tax (by reducing sugary drink consumption) but also aim to raise revenue (which is sometimes designated for specific purposes; e.g. the revenue from a soda tax in Philadelphia is allocated to early childhood education and community programmes). To give another example, efforts to open new grocery stores in underserved neighbourhoods aim to promote healthier eating by providing the community with healthier food, but also to create jobs and spur economic revitalization. We should expect that many healthy eating efforts will have multiple aims, only one of which is to make eating healthier; in fact, designing healthy eating efforts that have multiple aims has been explicitly embraced as sound strategy to overcome political obstacles to obesity efforts, since efforts with multiple aims (healthy eating, food security, environmental sustainability, youth empowerment, etc.) will attract broader coalitions of support (Barnhill et al. 2018).

Even when a healthy eating effort aims to make the target population healthier, the effort's *ultimate* aim may not be to improve 'the welfare, good, happiness, needs, interests or values' of the target population. Instead, it may be to reduce healthcare costs associated with diet-related illness, other economic costs (e.g. lower productivity amongst employees with diet-related illness), or other social costs of illness (e.g. the economic and psychological costs of illness for family caretakers). Advocacy for obesity prevention efforts does often emphasize the high healthcare costs associated with obesity, perhaps suggesting that reducing these healthcare costs is a major aim of obesity prevention efforts (e.g. IOM 2012). Indeed, some observers of public health have argued that in the US context, it is not uncommon for defenders of public health policies to dodge the charge of paternalism by emphasizing that the policies reduce the social costs of illness. However, this dodge may sometimes be disingenuous; policies might actually be animated by the intention to improve people's lives by making them healthier, but this intention is masked in order to preempt the charge of government paternalism (Bayer 2007; Colgrove and Bayer 2005).

Where does this leave us? To be fair to concerns about paternalism, we should assume that healthy eating efforts *do* have the aim of promoting healthy eating in order to advance individuals' welfare, though this may not be their only aim. Thus, in this chapter we assume that healthy eating efforts have paternalistic aims (at least towards some people) and consider objections to them as such.[1]

Let's turn now to our second query: Are healthy eating efforts based on the kinds of negative judgements that bother Quong? What *are* the judgements about efforts' targets that underlie these efforts, and are these negative judgements of the sort that bothers Quong?[2] Consider two different judgements that, plausibly, may underlie some healthy eating efforts:

---

[1] Ultimately, though, in Chapter 7 we propose a process of public justification of healthy eating efforts that does not assume that such efforts are paternalistic; they can in principle be justified either as paternalistic policies that help align people's dietary patterns with their life plans and conceptions of the good, or they can be justified as non-paternalistic policies on other grounds, e.g. because they advance the common good or equality of opportunity. What matters most, we will explain, is that such policies are justified based on a reasonable balance of political values.

[2] We put to the side healthy eating efforts that merely aim to inform the target population and are based in the judgement that they lack relevant information about food, nutrition, or health, and lack this information through no fault of their own. An example would be a law requiring food labels to include certain kinds of nutrition information (but not requiring that this information be presented in a graphic, compelling, or otherwise motivational way). Insofar as such policies are based on the judgement that the target population lacks relevant information through not fault of their own, they do not raise Quong's concerns, and we can put them to the side. However, if a labelling scheme—such as a food warning label presenting nutrition information in a graphic or 'scary' way—is motivated by the view that consumers have nutrition information but fail to be properly motivated by it, then this labelling scheme presumably would raise Quong's concerns.

i.   People reliably make decisions about food and manage particular situ-
     ations in a way that will effectively advance their welfare, interests,
     values, or life plans. However, in some contexts and for some people,
     eating in a less healthy way is what advances their welfare/life plan,
     given the costs of healthier eating and the benefits (hedonic, social, aes-
     thetic, cultural, etc.) of less healthy eating. Thus, healthy eating policy
     should aim to reduce the costs of healthier eating for the target pop-
     ulation (or increase the costs of less healthy eating), in order to make
     healthier eating the option that advances their welfare/life plan/etc.

ii. The policy's target population is apt, within contemporary food envir-
     onments, to engage in irrational eating behaviour or eating behaviour
     that does not effectively advance their welfare/life plan/etc.

Consider (i). Plausibly, this judgement underlies some healthy eating
efforts, i.e. those that try to decrease the costs (time, money, effort) of
healthier eating. Such efforts include subsidizing the purchase of healthier
foods by participants in food assistance programmes, efforts to make community gardens more widely available and accessible, and efforts to increase
geographic access to healthier foods (programmes to get corner stores to
offer healthier items, to get grocery stores to open in underserved areas, etc.).
Plausibly (i) also underlies efforts to increase the costs of less healthy eating,
such as taxes (e.g. sugary drink taxes) as well as programmes and policies
reducing the availability or prevalence of less healthy food (e.g. limits on the
density of fast-food restaurants and efforts to change which beverages and
foods are stocked in vending machines in schools and workplaces).

For both kinds of efforts, it is plausible that they are rooted in a judgement
like (i), that people reliably eat in ways that advance their welfare/life plan/
etc., but *healthier* eating often does not advance the welfare/life plans/etc.
of the target population given how costly healthy eating is for them relative
to less healthy eating. So understood, these efforts aim to reduce the actual
costs (economic or otherwise) of healthier eating, or to increase the actual
costs of less healthy eating, in order to make healthier eating the course of
action that is actually best for the target population. If this is the case, these
efforts do not rest on a judgement that the target population cannot effectively advance their own welfare or life plans; on the contrary, they are based
on the judgement that people respond rationally to economic incentives
and disincentives (more precisely, that people reliably respond to changes in
the money/time/effort costs of eating in ways that advance their welfare/life

plans/etc.). These efforts, so understood, are therefore not based on the kind of negative judgement that bothers Quong.

Next consider (ii), another judgement that may, plausibly, underlie some healthy eating efforts: the policy's target population is apt, within contemporary food environments, to engage in irrational eating behaviour or eating behaviour that does not effectively advance their welfare/life plans/etc. Broadly speaking, public health advocates, researchers, and officials sometimes defend healthy eating efforts by casting eating behaviour as not-fully-voluntary, uninformed, or irrational behaviour (as discussed in Chapters 1 and 2). Some proponents of healthy eating efforts argue that highly palatable foods undermine our ability to self-regulate our consumption, e.g. because they stimulate the reward system of the brain, motivating us to eat them again and again (Kessler 2009, pp. 14–15, 29; Roberto et al. 2015). They point to research on 'mindless eating' showing that food consumption is 'cued' by large serving sizes and other features of the food environment (Wansink 2007). This body of research has been taken to show that rather than deciding how much to eat based upon hunger or energy needs or pleasure, we seem to simply eat more when we are served more, in ways unbeknownst to ourselves and outside of our control.[3] There is also work on the addictiveness or quasi-addictiveness of highly palatable foods, which is cited in defence of healthy eating efforts (e.g. work on the addictiveness of sugar is sometimes cited in support of taxes on sugary drinks) (DiLeone et al. 2012; Volkow et al. 2013; Ziauddeen and Fletcher 2013). Furthermore, there is work discussing ways in which eating behaviour is systematically irrational (Conly 2013a; Sunstein 2014).[4]

Taken as a whole, this work paints a picture of eaters as often engaged in irrational and even not-fully-voluntary food consumption. Healthy eating efforts, then, can be seen as responding to and trying to correct this food consumption. To give a specific example, when the NYC Department of Health

---

[3] Note that some of this research, led by Brian Wansink, has been retracted. The scientific integrity of this body of research has been called into question. But that is not relevant to the point being made here, which is that *this kind* of research, when scientifically sound, can be used to explain and justify healthy eating efforts.

[4] For a discussion of cognitive biases and paternalistic policy, see also Trout (2005). These cognitive biases, to identify just a few, include the following: overconfidence in our own judgements; status quo bias, in which we attach greater value to the status quo than alternative courses of action that would otherwise be preferred; anchoring, in which background information influences judgements—anchoring them to an arbitrary point—even though it is irrelevant; and framing effects, in which choices are sensitive to how a problem is framed, even when the substance of the choices remains constant across framings.

and Mental Hygiene (2012) proposed a limit on the size of sugary drinks via the aforementioned 'soda ban', it pointed to research showing that individuals consume more when they are given larger servings:

> Larger portions lead to increased consumption and calorie intake. When people are given larger portions they unknowingly consume more and do not experience an increased sense of satiety. In one study, people eating soup from self-refilling bowls ate 73% more, without perceiving that they had eaten more or feeling more full. The same holds true with beverages. When served more fluid ounces of a beverage, people drink more without decreasing the amount of food they eat or experiencing a difference in 'fullness' or thirst.

Thus, the proposed policy limiting sugary drink size may have been based on the judgement that beverage consumption is not fully voluntary or is irrational. If healthy eating efforts are based on the view that the target population will behave involuntarily or irrationally in the absence of the policy, then they *are* based on the kind of negative judgement that bothers Quong—i.e. a negative judgement about people's ability to make the right decisions or manage particular situations in a way that will effectively advance their welfare, life plans, etc. Though Quong does not consider healthy eating efforts in particular, presumably he would object to such efforts on these grounds.

However, we would like to point out, the judgement that people will behave involuntarily or irrationally in some food environments need not be rooted in a negative judgement of people as practical reasoners. Rather, situationally irrational eating behaviour is often framed as a result of 'obesogenic' environments that undermine to some extent the individual's ability to regulate her food consumption (Brownell et al. 2010; Egger and Swinburn 1997; Schwartz and Brownell 2007). Obesity is a *normal* response to an *abnormal* environment, it is claimed. The problem is not with the people, who are behaving 'normally'; the problem is with the 'abnormal' environment. Thus, while it might be true that people are unable to manage contemporary food environments in a way that will effectively advance their welfare, life plans, etc., this is not because their practical reasoning is deficient in any notable way; it is because food environments undermine practical reasoning in normal humans.

In addition, the judgement that people behave irrationally in many contemporary food environments or contexts need not rest on the judgement that people lack the more general capacity to form a conception of the good and enact a life plan that aligns with that conception.[5] Nor need these efforts deny that people generally have the capacity to identify a dietary pattern that advances their life plan and aligns with their conception of the good. Rather, the assumption underlying these efforts could be the much narrower one that people do not *always* conform to the dietary pattern that would best advance their life plans and/or that they do not do so *in all food environments*. In other words, there might be healthy eating efforts based on this set of views:

ii'. The target population can in principle reliably identify dietary patterns that advance their life plans and align with their conceptions of the good. However, the policy's target population is apt, within certain contemporary food environments, to engage in irrational eating behaviour that is misaligned with those dietary patterns.

Quong, as we interpret him, would object to such policies, since they are rooted in the judgement that people will act irrationally in particular situations. Remember that Quong (2011, p. 101) adopts the Rawlsian requirement that governments are 'to act in accordance with principles that are consistent with, and give expression to, this conception of citizens as free and equal', and that this requires treating citizens as if they have the capacity for a conception of the good, which is 'the capacity to form, to revise, and rationally to pursue a conception of one's rational advantage or good' (pp. 100–101). Quong argues that when governments are motivated by the judgement that citizens act irrationally, this is a failure to treat citizens in the requisite way.

In our view, Quong's construal of the Rawlsian requirement is problematic and should be rejected since it does not allow for the interplay between environments and practical reasoning, and for the ways in which environments can undermine practical reasoning situationally. The liberal ideal that governments should treat people as free and equal should not be construed as requiring governments to assume—contrary to ample empirical evidence—that individuals act rationally in pursuit of their conception of the good in

---

[5] Jason Hanna (2018, pp. 82–83), in an illuminating defence of paternalism, critiques Quong's argument and makes a general version of the point we are making here: '[T]here is little reason to think that paternalistic intervention treats people as though they lack Rawls's second moral power. Such intervention may treat people as if they (or a sufficient number of them) are unlikely to exercise the second moral power in a maximally prudent way'. Correctly judging that someone sometimes acts imprudently does not amount to denying that they have the general capacity to form, to revise, and rationally to pursue a conception of their good.

all situations. This puts us in broad agreement with other work arguing that governments do not treat citizens disrespectfully when they accurately appraise citizens' rational abilities and design policies in light of predicted irrational behaviour (Conly 2013a; Hanna 2018).

4.5. What does it mean for healthy eating efforts to treat people as free and equal?

How, then, should we unpack the liberal ideal that governments should treat people as free and equal? If we accept that treating people as free and equal requires treating them as having the capacity to form, to revise, and to pursue a conception of their good, what exactly does this require? What kinds of views about citizens are incompatible with this requirement? And in the specific context of healthy eating efforts, what kinds of assumptions and judgements are consistent and inconsistent with this requirement?

Healthy eating efforts would run afoul of the requirement to treat people as having the capacity to form, to revise, and to pursue a conception of their good if they were based on the view that the target population has the wrong conception of the good, e.g. because they do not value health enough or appreciate the role of healthy eating or health in a good life. We argue, furthermore, that in the context of healthy eating efforts, recognizing people as having the capacity to form, to revise, and to pursue a conception of their good requires the following:

a. Recognizing and respecting people's diverse conceptions of health and the different value they place on health and on eating.
b. Recognizing people as being able to form and to pursue a life plan that aligns with their conception of the good.
c. Recognizing that food and eating play different roles in different people's life plans. Eating is a source of nutrition and health, but also has social, economic, and personal value and disvalue of various sorts. A less healthy dietary pattern could be the right trade-off for someone to make, given her life plan.

Doing (a)–(c) requires seeing eating not just as a source of nutrition and health but as having various kinds of (dis)value and recognizing the many roles that food and eating have in life plans (as we discuss in Chapter 1).

Food and eating are instrumental to survival, nutrition, short-term physical well-being (e.g. having energy), and long-term health and longevity. They can cause positive subjective experiences (e.g. pleasure, comfort, stress relief, satiation), and these positive subjective experiences have psychological benefits. Food and eating are also instrumental to social goods and social ends; e.g. eating together, cooking for one another, sharing food, and having a common cuisine can function to build and maintain social relationships.

But just as food experiences and dietary patterns can be a central part of our life plans, or instrumental to enacting those life plans, so too food experiences and dietary patterns can undermine the achievement of our life plans. Our dietary patterns can undermine our health, and thereby undermine our ability to enact our life plans. But healthier eating, too, can undermine the enactment of our life plans, due to the money, time, and effort spent on it. For example, spending time at the end of a busy workday making a home-cooked dinner for your children can leave no time to help them with their homework, get them to bed on time, or play with them. Healthy eating can have social costs, because it can reduce conviviality, increase interpersonal tension, and preclude meaningful shared experiences that involve less healthy eating. (See Chapter 1 for more discussion of these issues.)

Because food and eating have so many different kinds of value, there are conflicts and trade-offs. For example, the way you feed your family (e.g. making healthy home-cooked meals) could help you to achieve health-related ends and goals for you and your family, while being stressful and a source of tension and disagreement, thereby undermining other ends, such as family harmony. Which trade-offs are the (subjectively) best ones to make depends upon your ends, and how these ends fit into your life plan—the longer-term, stable, structured plan for a life.

The designers and advocates of healthy eating efforts should be alert to these various ways in which eating and food have value and disvalue, and not pay short shrift to the potential economic, social, and personal disvalue of healthy eating (Mayes and Thompson 2014; Resnik 2010). Policy designers need to recognize that people face different trade-offs around food because of the different practical circumstances of their lives (i.e. whether eating healthfully requires the sacrifice of other valuable ends depends upon economic and social circumstances). They need to recognize that which trade-offs are the best ones for someone to make depends upon their ends and life plans. And, lastly, they need to recognize that people have different ends because they have different life plans, rooted in different underlying conceptions of the good life. This is simply the result of 'reasonable disagreement', as defined by Rawls (see Chapter 2). Such disagreement is not irrational but the 'result of the normal functioning of human reasoning under reasonably favorable conditions' (Quong 2018).

We have suggested that recognizing people as having the capacity to form, revise, and rationally to pursue a conception of the good requires recognizing and respecting their different conceptions of health and the different values they place on health and eating. It also requires acknowledging that eating plays various different roles in people's life plans, and that less healthy eating experiences and less healthy dietary patterns may be the best course of action for some.

To put this recognition into practice, when particular healthy eating efforts are envisioned, it is important to consider how those particular efforts may affect the target population in the context of their lives and life plans.

4.6. Conly's defence of paternalism and the perfectionism objection

In this section, we consider a view that has interesting points of connection with ours: Conly's (2013a) defence of coercive paternalism. Conly argues in favour of paternalistic government policies, including *coercive paternalism* that eliminates choices or mandates certain actions (e.g. laws banning the sale of cigarettes or limiting portion sizes in fast-food restaurants). She argues that when people engage in irrational behaviour that is an ineffective means to accomplish their long-term ends, it can be justifiable for the government to interfere to change their behaviour so that they take effective means to their ends.

Consumption of unhealthy foods, Conly argues, is often this kind of irrational behaviour—irrational behaviour that undermines people's accomplishment of their long-term ends. An unhealthy dietary pattern undermines someone's health, and by undermining her health and shortening her life, an unhealthy dietary pattern can undermine her achievement of her long-term ends—both the long-term end of being healthy and staying alive, and all her other ends that require health and continued life.

According to Conly (2013a, p. 164), '[w]e want longer lives and we want good health, both as ends in themselves and as means to doing everything else we want to do'. She writes:

Generally, public health measures are intended to help people achieve what in fact they most want, in the long term, and most people want to live a long healthy life, both for its own sake, and because they also want to have other things of which they can have more if they live long healthy lives—social relationships, achievements or just time spent in pure enjoyment. (Conly 2013b, p. 241)[6]

Even though we want good health and long lives, we often act irrationally in ways that undermine our health; eating is a prime example. Conly (2013b, p. 242) gives this vivid description of how eating can fail to be rational:

To some extent, this phenomenon is familiar to us through introspection: we plan not to eat fattening food, but once we stand inside the bakery, what we do may be different. Our way of thinking about the decision changes, so that we start to think that, for example, it is ok because the circumstances in this case are special, and in the future we will never, ever, eat a piece of frosted triple layer cake again; or that because cholesterol has not killed us yet, it will not kill us in the future; or that we are not as likely as other people to suffer the illnesses that obesity brings on. It is not that we have changed our minds about what our goals are, and have decided that the taste of cake outweighs the advantages of health and long life. That could happen, but it is a different kind of case. For most of us, once we have wiped the last of the buttercream off our chins, we realize that we made a mistake, and wish we had not acted as we did.

Conly (2013a, pp. 162–69) specifically discusses and defends portion control policies—policies limiting the size of portions offered in restaurants, which prevent people from ordering large portions—as an instance of justifiable government paternalism. Portion control policies would address a feature of the food environment that causes irrational behaviour, namely larger portion sizes that cue us to eat more, even when eating more subverts our long-term goals. By helping us to be healthier, these policies would help us achieve our long-term goals.

---

[6] A similar point is made by Hanna (2018, pp. 91–92), according to whom '[e]veryone, regardless of his more comprehensive conception of the good life, can acknowledge that early death and disease are to be avoided, and everyone can thus recognize that health-based considerations provide at least some reason in favor of anti-tobacco laws. More generally, defenders of paternalism often appeal to widely recognized neutral goods such as health, longevity, financial security, psychological well-being, and increased opportunity'.

Conly admits that when policies interfere with people's choices or actions, this may amount to a failure to respect the person's autonomy. But, she argues, this is not a failure to respect *the person*. Respecting the person, according to her, does not require pretending that she is a rational agent who is well-suited to make all decisions for herself; instead, it means respecting her long-term goals and helping her meet them. Conly (2013b, p. 242) writes:

> [I]t does not degrade us, as humans, to accurately assess our abilities. I am not degraded if I am told that I have no future in the NBA, as this is entirely correct . . . it just is not degrading to acknowledge that we do not have certain abilities we would like to have, and might have thought we did have. Pretending that we are competent in ways we are not is no foundation for respect.

We are in agreement with Conly on this point. Conly argues, furthermore, that coercing people does not disrespect them when you are coercing them into accomplishing their own ends:

> [I]t looks as if coercing people to do what is good for them, by their own lights, seems to respect their values rather than to disrespect them: we take seriously what they most want, and help them avoid the pitfalls that temptation, or other sources of poor means-end thinking, can bring them to. Coercive intervention—making them to do the right thing—helps them instantiate their own values, by preventing the (admittedly voluntary) actions that are contrary to those values. (p. 241)

Importantly, Conly only supports paternalism that helps people accomplish *their own* ends or goals (which is known as *weak paternalism* or *means paternalism*, as opposed to *strong* or *ends paternalism*; e.g. see Dworkin 2020). Conly (2013a, p. 43) argues for paternalism 'in cases where people's choices of instrumental means are confused, in a way that means they will not achieve their ultimate ends'. But she rejects paternalistic action that overrides or usurps people's own ends: 'I do not argue that there are objectively good ends, or objectively rational ends, or ends objectively valuable in any way, which everyone should be made to pursue' (p. 43). Since limiting portion sizes helps people achieve their own ends by improving their health, it is not imposing one set of values upon everyone or imposing alien values upon anyone, in Conly's view. Rather, portion control policies help everyone achieve their own ends and live in accordance with their own specific values.[7]

To be clear, Conly does not support any and all coercive paternalism that helps people achieve their own ends. Rather, she identifies four conditions that coercive paternalism must meet in order to be ethically justified: the activity to be prevented on paternalistic grounds is opposed to the individual's long-term ends; the coercive measures employed are effective; the benefits of using coercive measures are greater than the costs; and the coercive measures are the most efficient way to prevent the activity (Conly 2013a, pp. 150–51).

4.6.1. Pugh's criticism: Conly's view is back-door perfectionism

In his commentary 'Coercive Paternalism and Back-Door Perfectionism', Jonathan Pugh (2014) has objected to Conly's argument that coercing people into improved health helps them achieve their own ends and live in accordance with their own values. Pugh accepts that health is a near-universal value: nearly everyone values health. But people can value other things that sometimes conflict with health, such as pleasure. And people weight these valued things differently; e.g. though you and I both value pleasure and health, I may attach relatively more weight to health than you do. For example, I value excellent health, and value pleasure insofar as that is consistent with excellent health. However, you value intense pleasure, and value good health insofar as that is consistent with intense pleasure. Behaviour that is consistent with my weighting of health vs. pleasure may not be consistent with your weighting of health vs. pleasure. Thus, paternalistic policies meant to improve our health can impose alien *weightings* of values upon

---

[7] Hanna argues that it is important to distinguish between two potential interpretations of Conly's argument. On one interpretation, which he calls 'the current desire-fulfillment account', means-related paternalism involves 'the fulfillment of the target's *current* desires, or provides him with what he most wants *now*' (Hanna 2018, p. 106, original emphasis). On another interpretation, 'the overall desire-fulfillment account', means-related paternalism promotes 'the overall fulfillment of the target's desires over the course of his whole life' (p. 106). According to Hanna, the former interpretation is not plausible, since paternalistic interventions are often unlikely to provide people with what they want now. But the latter interpretation, Hanna argues, is also problematic, since it presupposes that every person wants to maximize the fulfilment of their desires over the course of their lives (something means-paternalism helps them to do). That assumption, according to Hanna, is implausible and seems to betray an underlying form of ends-paternalism.

us, even if health is not an alien value and these policies are not imposing alien values upon us.[8] This is an instance of government perfectionism.

Therefore, if a portion control policy (i.e. a policy that limits portion sizes in order to reduce consumption of certain foods and improve health) is going to be defended as *weak* or *means paternalism*—i.e. as a policy that helps individuals achieve their own ends or goals—defenders are committed to something like this claim: individuals value the improvement in health likely to be achieved by the portion control policy more than they value whatever consuming larger portions would do for them (e.g. provide pleasure), and thus the portion control policy causes people to behave more in accordance with their values. Opponents like Pugh could argue that we cannot make this assumption; while it is probably true that some (or even many) people value the improved health more than the additional pleasure (or whatever else they get from the consumption that is being prevented), it is not plausible that *everyone* values health more. So the portion control policy does not help everyone behave in accordance with their own values and ends.

Thus it is an uphill battle to defend policies limiting access to unhealthy food as policies that help everyone (or nearly everyone) accomplish their long-term ends or behave in accordance with their values. For these policies to be defended as paternalistic policies, they will need to be defended as *strong/ends* paternalism, rather than *weak/means* paternalism, or as policies that are means paternalism vis-à-vis some people, but not paternalistic at all (in the sense of *means paternalism*) vis-à-vis those unfortunate others whose welfare is diminished by the policies. Thus, insofar as these policies are intended to help everyone better accomplish their (alleged) long-term ends, they do seem to be imposing one set of values upon everyone, even though not everyone shares these values. If healthy eating efforts are intended to help everyone accomplish their (alleged) long-term ends, they do seem guilty of a kind of perfectionism.

4.6.2. Partial means paternalism

But do healthy eating efforts intend to help everyone (or nearly everyone) become healthier and thereby better accomplish their long-term ends? These

---

[8] In his defence of paternalism, Hanna (2018, p. 92) presents this objection to paternalism in the following way: '[E]ven if all reasonable people can agree *that* something is valuable, they may (reasonably) disagree about *how* valuable it is relative to other goods'. Likewise, Simon Clarke (2006, p. 119) argues that 'the state may act paternalistically to provide neutral goods only when doing so does not override the [target's] ranking of [neutral] goods according to his conception of the good'.

efforts do not necessarily aim to improve the health of the entire affected population; they may aim to improve the health of just some people in that population. And when efforts aim to improve people's health, they may not aim to improve their health in order to help them accomplish their own ends or better enact their life plans. Rather, as discussed earlier, public health policies and programmes may aim to improve people's health in order to reduce healthcare costs and thereby promote the common good. These are aims that do not involve helping people to accomplish their own ends.

Even when public health policies and programmes *do* aim to improve health so as to help people accomplish their own ends, they need not be rooted in the assumption or judgement that everyone affected by the policy will be helped in this way. That is, healthy eating efforts can be a kind of *partial means paternalism*: they can aim to promote healthy eating in some portion of the targeted population, with the recognition that this will help some people better accomplish their own ends but will not help other people and may even undermine their achievement of their own ends. With partially means-paternalistic policies, there are winners and losers: some people affected by the policy will be benefitted (i.e. the policy will help them accomplish their own ends), and some people will not be benefitted and may even be harmed.[9]

Assuming that partial means paternalism is a plausible construal of healthy eating efforts, and that these efforts aim to help some (but not all) people better achieve their own ends, the question then is the following: is it perfectionist or otherwise objectionable to assume that *some* people's dietary patterns are not aligned with their long-term ends and life plans, and that healthier dietary patterns would help these people better achieve their long-term ends and enact their life plans? We think that this assumption is not objectionable, as we argued earlier.

However, another question about partial means paternalism presents itself: do such efforts treat the 'losers' in a justifiable way? If some people's existing dietary patterns are consistent with their life plans and their conceptions of the good, does this mean that policies steering those people into different, healthier eating are unacceptable? Does a policy that steers someone into healthier eating, when their existing (less healthy) dietary

---

[9] Hanna (2018, p. 98) makes a related point, i.e. that so-called paternalistic policies can have both paternalistic rationales (i.e. they will benefit some people affected by the policy) and non-paternalistic rationales.

pattern already aligns with their life plan and conception of the good, fail to treat them as having the capacity to form, to revise, and rationally to pursue a conception of the good? Not necessarily. As we will argue in the coming chapters, people are treated as free and equal so long as they are provided with an acceptable public justification for policies, and as long as this public justification involves a reasonable balance of shared political values. This may be consistent with enacting healthy eating efforts that are not aligned with some people's own life plans and conceptions of the good.

4.7. From anti-paternalism to public justification

Much work on public health policies and programmes, and healthy eating efforts in particular, focuses on paternalism. In this discussion, autonomy rights are prominent, as are concerns that paternalism is disrespectful or fails to treat people as free and equal when it judges that they are irrational or not capable of safeguarding their own interests. In this chapter, we have argued that some autonomy-based objections to paternalism assume perfectionism. We have also addressed the objection that paternalistic healthy eating efforts themselves are perfectionist, in the sense that they impose one set (or ranking) of values upon everyone. This debate therefore reveals that perfectionism may underlie both anti-paternalism and paternalism. As Steven Wall (2018, p. 174) cogently points out,

> [i]t is helpful to distinguish state paternalism that is perfectionist in-sofar as it is designed to promote or safeguard autonomy (Type 1 State Perfectionism) from state paternalism that is perfectionist insofar as it aims to steer people toward valuable options and away from disvaluable options in exercising their autonomous agency (Type 2 State Perfectionism). (see also Wall 1998, pp. 197–98)

Type 2 state perfectionism is what often underlies the view that governments can legitimately implement healthy eating efforts that compel or encourage people to live healthier lives, thus prioritizing health over other values.

We believe that both types of state perfectionism are politically illegit-imate. We say this not because we reject the value of either individual au-tonomy or health per se but because in either type of paternalism one value is overly prioritized, and *this* seems morally unjustified under conditions of

be nearly impossible standards to meet in a diverse society. What treating people as free and equal *does* demand in the context of healthy eating efforts is that people are provided with a public justification, and more specifically public reasons, for those efforts. Key to this kind of public justification is an honest account of the costs of healthy eating efforts rather than the assumption that healthy eating efforts always benefit people or help them align their eating with their life plans and conceptions of the good. Also key to this kind of public justification is the balancing of health and other values, rather than the prioritization of health over other values.[10]

We argue in Chapter 7 that what will facilitate the design of healthy eating efforts that can be publicly justified is a process of consultation, deliberation and policy design at the community level. Ideally, this process could be designed to serve multiple functions and have a range of benefits, such as gathering information about the costs and benefits of different foods and dietary patterns, and their personal, social, and cultural meanings, for the target population; identifying dietary changes that improve health without undermining individual, family, or community well-being in other ways and hopefully even improve well-being; exploring the disparate impact and (in)equity of potential healthy eating efforts; and designing healthy eating efforts that are more likely to be effective because they have been designed with community input and buy-in.

---

[10] Our view, in emphasizing that trade-offs must be recognized and health must be balanced against other values, is aligned with dominant approaches in applied public health ethics, according to which public health policies are ethically justifiable if they strike a reasonable balance between competing values, such as well-being, autonomy, and justice (Childress et al. 2002; Kass 2001). Our view is also aligned in some ways with that defended by Resnik (2014), who argues that there should be limits on coercive healthy eating policies, and that health must be balanced against other values.

5

Liberalism, Public Reason, and Healthy Eating Efforts

5.1. Introduction

We concluded the previous chapter by arguing that critically assessing healthy eating efforts within the framework of the paternalism/anti-paternalism debate is limiting. We suggested that such a critical assessment should instead be carried out from the perspective of a different framework, i.e. that of public justification and public reason.

The idea of public reason, which we briefly discussed in Chapter 2, is widely endorsed amongst contemporary liberal political philosophers. It was first introduced by John Rawls (2005a) in his *Political Liberalism*, and then adopted in various forms by many liberal thinkers over the past few decades. It still offers the grounds for one of the most influential liberal understandings of political legitimacy. Defenders of public reason argue that in order to be legitimate, political rules should be justified based on reasons that all citizens could accept at some level of idealization, i.e. public reasons. This claim, we saw in Chapter 2, is based on two key assumptions: first, contemporary liberal societies are fundamentally diverse; second, compelling citizens to obey political rules based on reasons they cannot accept entails failing to treat them as free and equal persons.

Public reason excludes from public justification controversial reasons grounded in religious, ethical, and philosophical doctrines not shared by all citizens in contemporary diverse societies. It includes, instead, reasons appealing to such rights and liberties as freedom of thought and conscience, freedom of religion, and freedom of association (Rawls 2005a, p. 223), which are central to the public political culture of liberal democratic societies, as well as those that appeal to 'the methods and conclusions of science when these are not controversial' (p. 224), or to 'plain truths now widely accepted, or available, to citizens generally' (p. 224).

Healthy Eating Policy and Political Philosophy. Anne Barnhill and Matteo Bonotti, Oxford University Press. © Oxford University Press 2022. DOI: 10.1093/oso/9780190937881.003.0006

In this chapter we ask the following question: when, if ever, are healthy eating efforts, i.e. policies and interventions aimed at promoting healthier eating, publicly justified and consistent with the idea of public reason? Our rationale for asking this question, and for adopting public reason as a framework, is the following. As we have already stressed at various points in the book, we believe that healthy eating efforts are both necessary and desirable in contemporary liberal societies. However, we also believe that the design of such efforts should be accompanied by a greater acknowledgement of the complex moral issues that surround them than is currently the case. The paternalism/anti-paternalism debate does not capture this complexity. Public reason offers a more promising framework: first, it seriously takes into account the fact of reasonable pluralism that characterizes contemporary liberal societies; second, it allows a range of political values to enter into consideration; and, third, it can help us to make sense of the complex empirical, epistemic, and moral issues that surround healthy eating efforts within a unified framework.

At this point we would like to make two important clarifications. First, unlike other authors who are concerned only with coercive healthy eating efforts (e.g. Rajczi 2008), we follow Colin Bird (2014) and assume that the ideal of public reason applies to both coercive and non-coercive legislation, therefore also to non-coercive healthy eating efforts. These include, e.g., healthy eating messaging campaigns, nutrition labelling legislation, efforts to make healthy food more widely available, and food bans that apply only to certain contexts (e.g. schools). These efforts are not (entirely) coercive; e.g. they do not render unhealthy food much harder to find or to procure. Second, we also assume, following Quong (2004), that the constraints of public reason apply to all legislation and not only to "'constitutional essentials" and questions of basic justice' (Rawls 2005a, p. 214). Rawls himself sometimes seems to endorse this approach (e.g. p. 215). This point is important since many healthy eating efforts are not related to constitutional and basic justice issues (though, as we will see, some are).

Our analysis proceeds as follows. First, we offer an account of various ways in which reasonable pluralism is relevant to a discussion of public reason and healthy eating efforts. We discuss the existence of different conceptions of health, different levels of priority assigned to health as opposed to other values, and different kinds of social and cultural importance assigned to eating practices. We then critically assess the implications of major conceptions of public reason, i.e. 'shareability', 'intelligibility', and 'accessibility' (Vallier 2014), for the public justifiability of healthy eating efforts. We do not intend to defend any of these conceptions per se but only assess whether any of them, as currently found in the literature, is consistent with healthy eating efforts. We conclude that healthy eating efforts are compatible with public reason only if one endorses an 'accessibility' conception according to which policies are publicly justified if they are based on reasons grounded in shared epistemic and moral evaluative standards, and as long as such reasons reflect a reasonable balance of political values and do not overly prioritize or neglect any of these values. The majority of healthy eating efforts, we claim, would not be publicly justified based on the main versions of the 'intelligibility' conception found in the literature, nor would they be publicly justified based on the 'shareability' conception.

5.2. Reasonable pluralism, health, and eating practices

In contemporary societies, people endorse different conceptions of health. Health may be understood, e.g., as the absence of illness, the ability to exercise autonomy and function in society, a form of wellness that includes spiritual well-being and interpersonal harmony, or as encompassing '[p]leasure, resilience, belonging and well-being' (Mayes and Thompson 2014, p. 165; see also Backett et al. 1994; Davis et al. 1992; Hughner and Kleine 2004; Lawton 2003; McKague and Verhoef 2003). Health is commonly understood to include mental health, but does it include psychological well-being more generally? Does it include social functioning? There are points of sharp disagreement, amongst both scholars and laypeople, about how health should be understood. For example, should any form of disability be seen as a state of reduced health that we have a collective reason to prevent, as many assume? Or are many disabilities not appropriately seen as states of reduced health, or even states of reduced well-being, but instead as merely different (but not worse) bodily states (Barnes 1996)?

Despite the differing conceptions of health at play, it is tempting to say that they do converge on a point of agreement: diseases (at least of certain sorts) reduce health on all these conceptions. Diseases such as cancer, diabetes, and cardiovascular disease that cause suffering, increase mortality,

and lower lifespans do, plausibly, reduce health no matter one's specific conception of health. It might seem, therefore, that there is a shared, though
narrow, conception of health: health as the absence of illness (excluding
disabilities). We might therefore be hopeful that the aim of reducing rates
of disease is a public health aim consistent with all reasonable conceptions
of health.

But there is a wrinkle. Efforts to reduce disease rates may have various
costs. For example, an intervention might reduce rates of sexually trans-
mitted infections by reducing sexual contacts or motivating people to use
disliked forms of birth control. An intervention might reduce lung cancer
rates by discouraging smoking through efforts that socially marginalize and
stigmatize smokers, e.g. fear-based messaging or laws prohibiting smoking
within and near workplaces, schools, and restaurants (Stuber et al. 2008).
In the case of diet-related illnesses, healthy eating efforts might encourage
healthier eating and thereby reduce disease risk, but also have social and personal costs for individuals and groups. Consider, e.g., the healthy eating recommendation to fill half of one's plate with vegetables (Tarkan 2011). If a
parent follows this recommendation for herself and her family, this might
reduce their disease risk but might also contribute to greater stress and less
conviviality at mealtimes, as discussed in Chapter 1. If one's conception of
health includes social and psychological well-being, this dietary change
could reduce overall health (according to one's own conception of health)
even while reducing risk of disease. The net result of an intervention could
be to reduce an individual's health (on her broader conception of health),
despite reducing her risk of specific diseases and thus promoting health narrowly intended.

Another variation on this problem is that even if we could come up with
an uncontroversial (narrow) notion of health, we would still have to face the
fact that people attach different relative value to health (narrowly intended)
in relation to other values, and have different views about the right trade-offs
for themselves between health and other valued things (Pugh 2014). That is,
even if we overcame disagreement about the meaning of health, we could still
face disagreement regarding what the good life is. Even if people agreed on
a (narrow) conception of health, they would not all agree about the relative
importance of health as compared to other aspects (pleasure, sociality, etc.)
of a good life.

Eating practices (including habitually eating unhealthy food) can be
sources of pleasure for individuals and can be central to their life plans and

conceptions of the good for other reasons; e.g. they can have social and cultural importance, express significant social identities, and serve important roles in maintaining relationships. For example, an ethnographic study of low-income Latinx families found that consumption of unhealthy foods was experienced as an important part of some relationships—e.g. sharing sweet treats with a visiting father (Mulvaney-Day and Womack 2009). For these families, 'relationships are preserved and maintained through eating together. Identifying with another in a close family way requires eating the food they bring and that they eat' (p. 254).

Just as eating not very healthy food can be central (and contribute) to people's life plans and conceptions of the good, *healthier* dietary patterns can hinder them. For example, a study of 150 Black, white, and Latina mothers, already mentioned in Chapter 1, found that making a home-cooked meal (which is often recommended as a strategy to eat more healthfully) has significant downsides for many mothers: it requires a predictable work schedule, which not all parents have; it can take time away from other valuable experiences, such as helping a child with her homework; it takes foresight and planning, such as prepping vegetables during the weekend; and it requires navigating family members' different preferences (Bowen et al. 2014).

This and similar empirical research suggests that consumption of unhealthy food can often help promote and realize people's life plans and conceptions of the good in certain respects, while healthy eating—or what it takes to accomplish healthy eating, such as cooking—can be detrimental to them in certain respects (see also Barnhill et al. 2014; Mayes and Thompson 2014). There are significant trade-offs and we cannot assume that health is harmonized with all the other ends and values at stake—e.g. that giving children healthy food will be experienced as expressing love, or that eating a healthy home-cooked dinner together will improve rather than worsen family relationships in all circumstances. A child's bonds with their father, e.g., may not be fostered by eating a home-cooked meal together but rather by the fact that the father brings candy when he visits (Mulvaney-Day and Womack 2009, p. 254). There can be conflicts between healthy eating and various ends people have, and in a pluralistic society we should expect these conflicts to vary between individuals and between groups. These variable conflicts have implications for the public justification of healthy eating efforts, as we discuss in the next section.

5.3. Healthy eating efforts and public reason

Public reason, we have seen, is the idea that state laws and policies should be justified on the basis of reasons that all citizens could accept at some level of idealization despite their different conceptions of the good. Views of public reason developed in the literature vary in two ways that are relevant to our analysis. First, they vary with regard to which reasons should be allowed into the process of public justification. Second, they vary with regard to what it takes for a policy or law to be justified or defeated by the reasons that are allowed into public justification. For example, are policies publicly justified only if there are no public reasons that could be offered in objection to them (i.e. if no one can reasonably reject them based on public reasons)? Or are policies justified so long as there are public reasons in their favour, and the balance of political values that underlies them is reasonable, even if some members of the public reject that balance? We will see that defenders of the 'intelligibility' conception of public reason tend to endorse the former position, whereas defenders of the 'shareability' and 'accessibility' conceptions tend to embrace the latter.

But let's begin by examining what kinds of reasons should be allowed into the process of public justification. With regard to this aspect, Vallier (2014) offers a useful categorization of three main conceptions of public reason: intelligibility, shareability, and accessibility. These conceptions vary depending on the role assigned to reasons and evaluative standards. Evaluative standards, Vallier (2016, p. 602) explains, are 'a set of prescriptive and descriptive standards or beliefs that a member of the public takes to justify her reason affirmations and that enables her to order her moral and political proposals'.

According to the intelligibility conception of public reason, 'A's reason R_A is intelligible for members of the public if and only if members of the public regard R_A as epistemically justified *for A* according to *A's evaluative standards*' (Vallier 2014, p. 106, emphasis added). In other words, neither the reasons employed in public justification nor the evaluative standards that underlie those reasons need to be shared amongst all citizens in order for those reasons to be suitable for public justification.

According to the shareability conception, instead, 'A's reason R_A is shared with the public if and only if members of the public regard R_A as epistemically justified *for each member of the public*, including A' (Vallier 2014, p. 110, emphasis added). Unlike intelligibility, therefore, shareability demands that *both* reasons *and*, implicitly, the evaluative standards that underlie those reasons, are shared amongst all citizens in order for those reasons to be suitable for public justification.

Finally, according to the accessibility conception of public reason, a reason R_A can offer a suitable public justification for a law or policy if it is *accessible* to all citizens at the right level of idealization, i.e. if they 'regard R_A as epistemically justified *for A* according to *common evaluative standards*' (Vallier 2014, p. 108, emphasis added). As this definition suggests, accessibility offers a third way between intelligibility and shareability. While it does not demand that a reason be shared amongst all citizens in order for it to be suitable for public justification, it *does* require that any reasons put forward in public justification should be grounded in evaluative standards that are widely shared (rather than in evaluative standards that are endorsed by only one or a few specific person(s)).

These conceptions of public reason, as we will explain shortly, are not Vallier's creation but can be traced back to the works of various authors. However, the systematic character of Vallier's categorization offers a particularly useful theoretical framework for our analysis, and it is therefore to Vallier's work account that we will often refer.

5.3.1. Intelligible reasons and healthy eating efforts

The intelligibility conception of public reason is the one defended by Vallier himself as well as by Gaus (2010) and Gaus and Vallier (2009). This view, normally also referred to as the 'convergence' view of public reason (to be contrasted with 'consensus' approaches), has been criticized on different grounds. Some have argued, e.g., that it relies on a controversial relativist conception of justification (Quong 2011, pp. 261–73), while others have pointed out that it fails to provide citizens with a mutual assurance that they are truly committed to a political conception of justice in spite of their diverse conceptions of the good (Macedo 2010; Weithman 2010; but see the counterargument by Kogelmann and Stich (2016)). We set these critiques aside here.

What we would like to focus on, instead, is a third and, in our view, more powerful critique, i.e. the view that intelligibility allows most laws and policies, including healthy eating efforts, to be defeated by merely intelligible reasons (Vallier 2016, p. 603). Intelligibility is the most inclusive conception of public reason, in the sense that it includes the most reasons as public reasons. Since it does not require appealing either to shared reasons (shareability) or to shared evaluative standards (accessibility), it allows a significantly wider range of reasons (i.e. than shareability or accessibility) to enter the 'justificatory pool' (Vallier 2011, p. 372), i.e. the process of public justification during which public reasons are assessed and weighed against each other.

This, it should be pointed out, does not mean that intelligibility allows *any* reasons to enter the justificatory pool. First, not only the person who offers the relevant reason but also '*members of the public* . . . [must] regard R_A as epistemically justified for A according to A's evaluative standards' (Vallier 2014, p. 106, emphasis added). Second, under the intelligibility conception, a person '[must make] no gross epistemic error in affirming [a reason]' (p. 106), even if the latter is based on their own (non-shared) evaluative standards. Finally, intelligibility also involves moral constraints; e.g. it excludes reasons grounded in 'deeply egoistic' or 'sadistic and masochistic evaluative standards', which assume that people can be treated as means rather than ends (Vallier 2016, p. 610).

Even once we take into account these constraints, however, the reasons allowed into public justification by the intelligibility view may include those grounded in conceptions of health that rely on religious, supernatural, or folk explanations, or on other very controversial worldviews whose epistemic grounds and methods of enquiry are widely contested and not shared by those citizens who do not espouse such convictions. These and other reasons (which intelligibility allows but shareability and accessibility exclude, as we will show) may often defeat proposals for healthy eating efforts aimed at reducing people's risk of illness, if they conflict with the reasons that underlie those efforts (e.g. reasons based on a narrow conception of health and/or on the ranking of health thus intended above other values). In other words, the more permissive nature of intelligibility (compared to shareability and accessibility) is a double-edged sword when it comes to justifying healthy eating efforts: more reasons are allowed to justify these efforts, but more reasons are also allowed to defeat such efforts. In the words of Vallier (2016, p. 603, original emphasis) himself:

> [W]hile intelligible reasons are allowed into public deliberation, many other intelligible reasons may override the intelligible reasons that support

the law by defeating the law in question. In the absence of a successful justification, the default action is *state inaction*, which suggests that intelligibility will make state coercion much harder to justify. Intelligibility is permissive with respect to which reasons enter into public justification, but demanding about which reasons may eventually justify coercion.

More recently, Vallier (2019, p. 114) has acknowledged again this implication of intelligibility, recognizing that the 'anarchy objection', i.e. the view that '[if] everything is controversial . . . nothing is justifiable to all the reasonable' (Enoch 2015, p. 122), is 'a serious threat' (Vallier 2019, p. 115) to the intelligibility view.[1] Therefore, since intelligible reasons, according to one of the strongest advocates of intelligibility, can act directly as defeaters against the reasons that underlie many policies, and since intelligibility allows many more reasons into public justification than shareability or accessibility, it can be plausibly argued that intelligibility will rule out most healthy eating efforts.

It should be noted, however, that simply having intelligible reasons to *object* to a certain policy (e.g. a healthy eating policy) does not entail having intelligible reasons that *defeat* that policy. Existing defenders of the intelligibility view argue instead that in order for a law or policy to be deemed publicly unjustified, it must be shown that for at least some members of the public, based on their intelligible reasons, implementing such a law or policy would be worse than implementing *no law at all* in the relevant area (Gaus 2010; Vallier 2014, pp. 27–28). In response, it is plausible to argue that many members of the public in contemporary liberal democratic societies have intelligible reasons for considering healthy eating efforts worse than having no such efforts, even if they may be prepared to accept laws and policies in other areas, e.g. laws that protect freedom of speech or rights against bodily harm (Gaus 2010, Chap. 6). Indeed Gaus himself argues that under his conception of public reason, anti-smoking laws cannot be publicly justified since many citizens will have intelligible defeaters against the prioritization of health over pleasure that underlies such laws (p. 537).

Here it should be noted that sometimes those who oppose healthy eating efforts may accept other types of public health interventions, e.g. those that arise from collective action problems rather than being primarily aimed

---

[1] Vallier's attempt to answer this criticism seems to entail a move from intelligibility to accessibility (Bonotti 2020b).

at regulating people's behaviour. Take, e.g., vaccinations. Jason Brennan, a libertarian, argues that we have a moral duty not to take part in collectively harmful activities. Since vaccinations aim to prevent the spread of infectious diseases (a collective harm), it is therefore morally permissible for the state to compel people to vaccinate against such diseases (Brennan 2018). However, healthy eating efforts do not seem to present similar collective action problems. Therefore most libertarians, who are likely to endorse the intelligibility conception of public reason (insofar as they accept public reason at all), are likely to reject them. In conclusion, the intelligibility conception of public reason, as developed by its main defenders, Vallier and Gaus, does not seem to offer much scope for healthy eating efforts. In most cases, the presence of intelligible defeater reasons against such efforts amongst members of the public will result in state inaction in this area.

However, in spite of our criticism of intelligibility, we recognize that the latter can still play a role in public justification. More specifically, while not sufficient for public justification, intelligible reasons are necessary for what Rawls (2005a, pp. 386–87) calls *full* (as opposed to *pro tanto*) public justification. The former is realized only when citizens endorse political rules based on both public reasons and reasons grounded in citizens' diverse non-public conceptions of the good (which is to say, intelligible reasons). Furthermore, ensuring that intelligible reasons justify political rules is also important to generate the 'overlapping consensus' (Rawls 2005a) on a shared political conception of justice that for Rawls guarantees the stability of a political liberal order over time: only if citizens are able to endorse liberal political rules from their own particular perspectives, Rawls argues, will they be motivated to comply with them. Intelligible reasons can therefore be pragmatically important for healthy eating policy design. Finding justifications for healthy eating efforts that can 'speak to the heart' of people from different ideological and/ or religious backgrounds can help increase support for such efforts and increase their uptake and effectiveness.

5.3.2. Shareable reasons and healthy eating efforts

The shareability conception of public reason demands that a reason be admitted into public justification only if 'each citizen will affirm the reason *as her own* at the right level of idealisation' (Vallier 2014, p. 109, original emphasis). In other words, each citizen must accept the reason against the background of their *subjective motivational set* (Vallier 2011, p. 370, original emphasis), which includes one's beliefs and desires as well as 'dispositions of evaluation, patterns of emotional reaction, personal loyalties, and various projects' (Williams 1981, p. 102, cited in Vallier 2011, p. 387, note 11). A person's subjective motivational set may therefore include their beliefs and values associated with health and eating practices, e.g. beliefs regarding the value of conviviality and pleasure as they relate to eating, and the priority these should be assigned over health.

The shareability conception is defended, e.g., by Micah Schwartzman (2011, p. 378), for whom 'political justifications . . . must be based on shared or public reasons', and by James Bohman and Henry Richardson (2009), according to whom the idea of *potentially* acceptable shared reasons is not more sensitive to reasonable pluralism than that of *actually* accepted shared reasons, and therefore the latter is preferable.

Is shareability consistent with healthy eating policy? One might argue that it can be, if there is a conception of health that is shared by all citizens (at the right level of idealization). We saw earlier that a conception of health that equates it to the absence of illness may offer such a narrow and publicly shared conception. However, we also saw that even if we agree on a (narrow) definition of health, people with different conceptions of the good will still disagree on how to rank a healthier life (narrowly understood) in relation to other values. For example, even if it could be shown, for the sake of argument, that 'health is the absence of illness' is a neutral and uncontroversial definition of health, widely shared amongst scholars and laypeople within contemporary liberal democracies, it is likely that many citizens would rank the promotion of 'health as the absence of illness' lower than other values and goods related to eating, including pleasure, conviviality, or values associated with their cultural identity. More precisely, many citizens might rank additional reductions in their risk of illness (from eating more healthfully) lower than other values and goods that would be sacrificed in order to achieve a lower risk of illness (e.g. pleasure and conviviality). We also highlighted this problem when critically assessing Conly's paternalism in the previous chapter.

But the promotion of health via healthy eating efforts cannot be an end in itself. These efforts are normally grounded in the view that promoting health can help advance certain shared political values. Indeed, for Rawls (2005a, p. 228), citizens can enjoy their basic rights and liberties only if they also have access to a 'social minimum', i.e. a set of goods that helps them to fulfil their basic needs and thus protects them from such conditions as hunger or disease (Kaufman 2018, pp. 223–24). Furthermore, healthy eating efforts can be said to contribute to citizens' equality of opportunity, a natural extension of Norman Daniels's (2008) argument that equality of opportunity requires access to healthcare (since taking advantage of the opportunities available in a society requires a minimum level of health). Additionally, healthy eating efforts can help promote the well-being of individuals and enable them to enact their own life plans and conceptions of the good. Furthermore, they can help realize the common good, e.g. because a healthier society is economically more prosperous. More specifically, they can help reduce the social costs of poor health, including healthcare costs but also costs on the economy due to lower levels of productivity, as well as reduce the economic and psychological costs borne by the caretakers of sick people.

Yet, even though the realization of these values via healthy eating efforts would seem to be a widely appealing goal, the public justification offered in support of these efforts may not sufficiently take into account many citizens' motivational sets. Therefore, the question to be asked, from the perspective of shareability, is not whether members of the public share the same conception of health, or whether they share the view that health should be promoted in order to advance broadly shared political values such as basic rights and liberties or equality of opportunity. Instead, the key question is whether they would accept efforts that promote health to realize these values *even though these efforts conflict with their individual beliefs, desires, and loyalties.* It is plausible to assume that many citizens would not accept this kind of trade-off. For example, a ban on foods or drinks, or a sugary drink tax, might help decrease disease risk but also reduce the pleasure of those who enjoy consuming the relevant foods or drinks. For these citizens, arguing that such efforts aim to promote health and equality of opportunity will not count as a shared public reason since this way of promoting those values (which they may generally endorse) will conflict with their individual preferences and desires.

To give another example, imagine an intervention that works with mothers to encourage dietary change—e.g. by offering nutrition education and cooking classes that teach them how to cook healthy meals, and by offering them financial incentives if they make healthy home-cooked meals for their families several times each week. Let's zoom in on this example and imagine two scenarios.

First, imagine a mother for whom the policy is clearly impractical and in-convenient—e.g. a mother who is already extremely burdened, who cannot easily afford healthier food even when offered financial incentives, and whose family is very inconvenienced by the additional expense and stress. We can describe this healthy eating intervention as clearly inappropriate for her, simply in virtue of being impractical or very inconvenient. We could ex-pect agreement (or lack of reasonable disagreement) that the intervention is inappropriate *if targeted towards mothers like her*. But imagine a second scenario in which the intervention is targeted at other mothers, for whom the financial incentives enable buying healthier food, and for whom the in-tervention is not quite as burdensome, impractical, or inconvenient. In this scenario, we can imagine reasonable disagreement as to whether the costs are warranted by the potential health benefits. It is this kind of scenario that we are interested in here.

Suppose, e.g., that a mother does not think that cooking healthy home-cooked meals several nights a week is worth the costs, e.g. because this would create a more stressful home environment (because she would be more rushed in the evenings, and her kids would protest the new meals), and because her family would derive less pleasure and psychological com-fort from their food. In other words, she does not think she has reason to reduce their risk of diet-related illness (and thus increase their health-de-pendent opportunities) in this way, i.e. by changing her family's diet as advo-cated by the policy. Should we say that she shares the justification for the policy? Shareability, we have seen, demands that each citizen ought to ac-cept a reason against the background of their beliefs, desires and loyalties. Should we say that this mother shares the justification for the policy because she shares the aim of reducing her children's risk of diet-related illness? Or should we say that she does not share the justification for the policy because she does not share the aim of reducing their risk of diet-related illness *in this way*? The latter seems more plausible.

On the one hand, we might be tempted to say that the policy has an aim (the aim of *reducing diet-related illness*) that is shareable. On the other hand, we might say that the policy does not have a shareable aim, because this aim is not simply reducing diet-related illness but rather *reducing diet-related ill-ness in this way*—a way that is in tension with this mother's beliefs and values. Furthermore, it seems that whichever way of reducing diet-related illness we opt for (e.g. if we replace diet-related health interventions with interventions encouraging mothers to exercise regularly and have their families do so), we are likely to encounter the same problems.

The more general point, therefore, is that appealing to the promotion of health as the absence of illness in support of healthy eating efforts (and health-promoting state interventions more generally), as a way of realizing broadly shared political values, would not count as a shared public reason for many citizens. This is because many citizens would rank reductions in illness and the advancement of those broadly shared values lower than other values and goods that they individually cherish, when such values and goods are threatened by healthy eating efforts.

At this point, a critic might insist that the aim of many healthy eating efforts, suitably specified, is shareable. A healthy eating programme or policy might improve the health and well-being of one segment of the population, while having no effect or a negative effect on another segment. After all, public health efforts normally 'aim to realise health benefits at a group or population level' (Dawson and Verweij 2007, p. 7) rather than at the individual level. This means that the aim of a given healthy eating effort, such as the aforementioned intervention targeting mothers, is not to reduce diet-related illness in this way *for everyone potentially reached by the policy*. Rather, more plausibly, its aim is to reduce diet-related illness in this way *for the population as a whole*. This is consistent with acknowledging that in order to achieve this goal the policy will actually benefit only some of the target audience while having no effect or a negative effect on others (although the policymaker cannot predict who will be affected in which way) (e.g. see Walker 2016). The critic could then argue that *this* aim, i.e. the aim of reducing diet-related illness at the population level, could be shared, even by those who are negatively affected by the policy qua individuals. Even if the overburdened and under-resourced mother cannot share the aim of reducing *her and her family's* risk of diet-related illness in this way, she could share the aim of reducing population-level risk in this way.

This objection, however, seems to presuppose a rather narrow understanding of what a person's subjective motivational set includes. More specifically, it would be misleading to limit the range of beliefs, desires, personal loyalties, etc. that a person has to those that concern only *their* (or *their family's*) well-being. Many people's beliefs, desires, and personal loyalties, indeed, concern not only their own (or their family's) well-being but also that of society as a whole. Many people have beliefs and personal loyalties associated with ethical, religious, or political worldviews that involve a vision of how society should be run, i.e. conceptions of the *common good* on the basis of which the well-being of the population as a whole should be promoted.

Setting aside clearly illiberal views—e.g. those that advance visions of the common good that involve harm or discrimination against members of certain groups—some of the visions of the common good consistent with liberalism, and which can be part of people's motivational sets, may still be in tension with the state's aim to reduce diet-related illness through efforts like our hypothetical intervention targeting mothers. Those who hold these visions of the common good might believe, e.g., that these interventions reinforce gender stereotypes according to which mothers have primary responsibility for the family's health or cooking meals for the rest of the family is the mother's role; or that they unduly encourage a lifestyle that prioritizes certain (family- and home-related) values over others; or that they put responsibility for healthier eating almost entirely on individual families, when there should be more shared social responsibility for healthier eating, e.g. by providing subsidies for prepared healthy meals or changing work and school schedules to reduce the inconvenience of home-cooking; or that public resources are limited, and promoting people's physical activity and sport, rather than spending money to subsidize healthier eating, would be a better way of reducing their risk of becoming ill. In other words, by shifting the debate from the individual to the population level, the tension between the reasons offered in support of a healthy eating effort and many people's subjective motivational set is still present.

Another example also illustrates this point. As discussed in previous chapters, public health officials and policymakers in several US states have proposed excluding sugary drinks and candy from the foods that can be purchased using food assistance—more specifically, using food assistance provided by SNAP, which is the largest food assistance programme in the US, offering assistance to 40 million people each year. A modest majority of participants in SNAP support excluding sugary drinks from it (Long et al. 2014). However, advocates for low-income people and anti-hunger advocates, and some members of the public, have raised ethical objections to excluding foods from SNAP. These exclusions are claimed to be infantilizing and demeaning, and to unfairly single out SNAP participants, amongst other concerns. These concerns have been voiced in the popular press and by advocates for low-income people (FRAC 2017a).

Some argue that rather than promoting SNAP participants' health by restricting their food choices, an ethically better way to promote their health would be by giving them additional food assistance with which to buy healthy foods. In other words, some people have ethical objections to the way in which SNAP exclusions promote healthy eating (by restricting the choices available to participants in this food assistance programme) even if they embrace the goal of promoting healthy eating. Here we see another example of the aim of a policy—to improve public health by restricting the choices available to SNAP participants when they use food assistance—not being shareable from the perspective of advocates for low-income people and anti-hunger advocates. In view of these problems, it can be concluded that one cannot be committed both to a shareability conception of public reason and to the implementation of healthy eating efforts.

5.3.3. Accessible reasons and healthy eating efforts

According to the accessibility conception of public reason, we have already seen, a reason R_A can offer a suitable public justification for a law or policy if it is *accessible* to all citizens at the right level of idealization, i.e. if they 'regard R_A as epistemically justified *for A* according to *common evaluative standards*' (Vallier 2014, p. 108, emphasis added). The accessibility conception is endorsed, e.g., by Robert Audi (2011, p. 70), who argues that

> adequate reasons . . . [do not need] to be shared by everyone. They need only be in a certain way accessible to rational adults: roughly, appraisable by them through using natural reason in the light of facts to which they have access on the basis of exercising their natural rational capacities.

Likewise, Rawls (2005a, p. 224) seems to endorse accessibility when he claims that reasons are public when they are grounded in 'guidelines of inquiry: principles of evidence of reasoning and rules of evidence' (see also Vallier 2014, p. 108).

Under the accessibility conception, healthy eating efforts could be publicly justified by reasons that appeal to shared evaluative standards. These may include, e.g., the methods and standards of the natural sciences. Importantly, unlike shareability, accessibility allows the use of some controversial reasons to justify political rules. These reasons may be controversial either because there is disagreement about their content and meaning amongst experts and/ or the general public (e.g. there is not a shared conception of health) or because they cannot count as reasons in the light of many citizens' motivational sets, as in the examples discussed in the previous section. For instance, even if not all citizens rank health defined as 'the absence of illness' above many or most of their other values, appealing to the promotion of health so defined as a way of, say, advancing equality of opportunity may still count for them as an accessible public reason that provides a public justification for the relevant healthy eating effort. Indeed those who invoke such a reason can appeal to the fact that the view that health is the 'absence of illness' is widespread in liberal societies. Even those who believe that health involves more than just the absence of illness are likely to agree that at the very least being healthy means not being ill. In other words, this narrow conception of health is one of those 'presently accepted general beliefs and forms of reasoning found in common sense' (Rawls 2005a, p. 224) which are part of the content of public reason. Furthermore, equality of opportunity is part of the content of public reason in a liberal democracy and constitutes one of its shared moral evaluative standards. In sum, accessibility allows policymakers to justify healthy eating efforts by appealing to reasons that may not be shared amongst the public, as long as these reasons are grounded in evaluative standards that are widely shared.

At the same time, accessibility rules out as sources of public reason, e.g., those conceptions of health that rely on religious, supernatural, or folk explanations, whose epistemic grounds and methods of enquiry are widely contested and not accessible to those citizens who do not espouse such convictions. In spite of these constraints, accessibility allows a much wider range of healthy eating efforts than shareability, since the latter excludes from public justification not only reasons grounded in controversial non-shared evaluative standards but also those that, while grounded in shared evaluative standards—e.g. 'health as the absence of illness'—are in tension with many people's subjective motivational sets.

But recall that we should consider not only the definition of health used in the public justification of healthy eating efforts but also the values that the promotion of health supposedly helps advance. Interventions that pursue health on an accessible notion of health (such as health as the absence of illness) may still pursue health in particular ways that some reject—e.g. the aforementioned hypothetical intervention with mothers which encourages behaviour change in ways that some mothers do not think are worth the cost, since they conflict with their beliefs and desires. Can we justify such interventions, which achieve health aims by imposing certain sacrifices and trade-offs, such as a trade-off between disease risk and pleasure, or between disease risk and family conviviality? Are such justifications available on the accessibility conception of public reason? We think that they are.

To understand why, however, it is necessary to unpack further the structure of public reason under the accessibility conception. Unlike with the shareability conception, simply stating that the public justification for a policy conflicts with one's motivational set is not sufficient to consider that policy publicly unjustified under the accessibility conception. But neither is it permissible, under this conception, to implement *any* policy as long as its justification appeals to shared political values. To understand this point, let's consider Rawls' account of public reason, the most influential in the literature. According to Rawls (2005a, p. 224), we have already seen, the shared evaluative standards on which accessibility relies include 'guidelines of inquiry: principles of evidence of reasoning and rules of evidence' (e.g. the scientific method). These epistemic evaluative standards, according to Rawls, are widely shared within liberal democratic societies. Alongside them, however, Rawls highlights how liberal societies also present various shared liberal political values, i.e.

> the values of political justice . . . [i.e.] the values of equal political and civil liberty; equality of opportunity, the values of social equality and economic reciprocity; and . . . values of the common good as well as the various necessary conditions for all these values. (p. 224)

These shared general values can be considered moral evaluative standards which, alongside the aforementioned epistemic evaluative standards, can help us to establish which healthy eating efforts are consistent with public reason.

More specifically, in order to enter the justificatory pool (i.e. the process of public reasoning), the reasons on which proposed efforts are grounded need to be accessible; i.e. they need to be grounded in shared guidelines of enquiry (epistemic evaluative standards) and factual evidence, and to contribute to the advancement of shared political values (moral evaluative standards). This rules out clearly illiberal reasons, i.e. reasons which, even if epistemically accessible, openly reject or deny basic liberal values such as basic rights and liberties or equality of opportunity (e.g. using sound scientific methods or tools to exterminate members of an ethnic minority). However, many reasons will be both epistemically accessible and consistent with shared political values. Nevertheless, each reason may present a different balance of shared values, which will be assessed during the process of public reasoning. That assessment will involve, e.g., establishing whether the way in which a scientifically sound conception of health is employed to justify certain healthy eating efforts overly favours certain shared values over others. This process is crucial since, as Rawls (2005a, p. 227) himself admits, 'not any balance of political values is reasonable'.

How does this apply, then, to the public justification of healthy eating efforts? Suppose that a healthy eating effort (e.g. banning foods high in sodium, limits on the portion sizes of fast-food entrees, interventions encouraging mothers to feed families more healthfully, etc.) is aimed at promoting 'health as the absence of illness' (a widely shared conception of health) in order to promote citizens' equality of opportunity (a broadly shared liberal political value): in order to have an equal opportunity to lead a life conforming with their conception of the good, people need at least a certain level of health (i.e. intended as the absence of illness), and thus healthy eating efforts can promote equality of opportunity. Suppose also that these efforts are aimed at promoting 'health as the absence of illness' (a widely shared conception of health) in order to reduce health costs from diet-related illness and thereby promote society's financial good, which contributes to the common good (also a broadly shared political value in liberal societies). These interventions, despite being grounded in accessible reasons (since they rely on scientific evidence and aim to promote broadly shared political values), might nonetheless fall afoul of the accessibility conception of public reason *if they overly prioritize* certain shared political values over others. For example, interventions encouraging mothers to cook home-cooked meals may promote health and equality of opportunity while also exacerbating the unequal division of domestic work between the genders, thereby contravening the ideal of gender equality (another broadly shared political value in liberal societies).

Likewise, central to political liberalism is the recognition that individual citizens have two 'moral powers', i.e. 'the capacity for a sense of justice' and 'the capacity to form, to revise, and rationally to pursue a conception of one's rational advantage or good' (Rawls 2005a, p. 19). The ability of citizens to exercise these moral powers is a shared political value in a liberal society (Rawls 2005a, p. 203). Therefore, if, while appealing to the promotion of health and equality of opportunity, the justification for a healthy eating effort overly neglects values that are central to some citizens' ability to exercise their conception of the good (e.g. pleasure and conviviality as they relate to eating), that will result in an unreasonable balance of political values.

Healthy eating interventions that overly prioritize certain political values over others and/or fail to sufficiently take into account the latter are not publicly justified under the accessibility conception since they are grounded in an unreasonable balance of political values. As Quong (2011, p. 207) points out, an argument advanced in public justification 'must represent a plausible [i.e. reasonable] balance of political values. An argument, even if based on a political and free standing value, fails to be a reasonable public justification if it does not plausibly address other political values that may be at stake'.

This has another important implication. One might argue that people can appeal to accessible reasons in order to reject healthy eating efforts, and that these reasons may act as defeaters and override accessible positive reasons in favour of such efforts, thus resulting in the same kind of state inaction in the area of healthy eating policy that, we argued, will normally result from the intelligibility conception of public reason. However, this is not the standard understanding of accessibility and, more generally, of consensus (as opposed to convergence) approaches to public reason defended in the literature.[2] Those who, like Rawls, Quong, and others, endorse consensus conceptions of public reason generally believe that as long as a law is justified based on a reasonable balance of political values, the fact that other citizens, based on a different but equally reasonable balance of political values, may object to that law will *not* count as a defeater against that law; i.e. it will not render that law publicly unjustified.

Quong (2011, p. 205) illustrates this point with the example of Tony and Sara, two members of the public who disagree regarding the issue of the hiring of priests in the Catholic Church. By appealing to the value of religious liberty, Tony believes that the Catholic Church should have the right to employ male priests only. By appealing to the value of non-discrimination in employment, Sara believes instead that the Catholic Church should be compelled to comply with laws against gender discrimination in employment and, therefore, to also employ female priests. According to Quong, since

---

[2] We set aside here the shareability conception as we have already shown that it is not suitable for publicly justifying healthy eating efforts.

both Tony and Sara are appealing to shared political values, they both offer publicly acceptable reasons for the conflicting policies that they respectively endorse. In this and similar cases, the key requirement is that those engaging in public reasoning offer a 'plausible balance of political values . . . [i.e. that] [e]ach argument recognizes that there are multiple political values at stake, and each offers a plausible explanation as to why one public value ought to be prioritized over the other in cases of this kind' (p. 209). Crucially, according to Quong, neither Tony's nor Sara's reasons constitute defeaters against each other's proposed policy.

This implies that an accessibility conception of public reason grounded in shared moral evaluative standards (i.e. shared political values) can be 'inconclusive' (Quong 2011, p. 209); i.e. it can allow many rivalling yet equally legitimate accessible reasons and, therefore, many rivalling yet equally legitimate policies grounded in those reasons. Even though any of these reasons (and the resulting policies) might be 'reasonably rejectable' (p. 209) by other citizens who endorse rivalling reasonable reasons, the key point is that such citizens could have in principle endorsed the reasons in support of the policy. The link between accessibility and inconclusiveness in Quong's example is due to the fact that 'Tony's argument is . . . based on a clearly identifiable political value [i.e. religious liberty] to which Sara is firmly committed' (p. 209), and vice versa. The presence of these shared political values (which, alongside many others, are endorsed by all reasonable persons in liberal democratic societies) is what renders Tony's and Sara's reasons accessible and results in the inconclusiveness of public justification. This also ensures that both Tony and Sara 'can understand and accept [each other's reasons] *in* [*his or*] *her capacity as a free and equal citizen,* even if [he or] she does not believe it is the best argument, or even if [he or] she believes it to be incorrect' (p. 209). Understood in this way, the reasonable balance of political values that is central to accessibility constitutes a kind of compromise amongst the deliberating parties (Lister 2007).

The same point could be expressed by drawing on Andrew Lister's (2013) 'reasons-for-decisions' approach to public justification. According to Lister, we can distinguish between a 'reasons-for-decisions' and a 'coercion' model of public justification. While the former demands only that members of the public agree on what reasons count as public by appealing to certain shared criteria (thus excluding, e.g., most religious reasons from public justification), the latter demands that they agree on what specific policies are publicly justified. The key point, for Lister, is that as long as people agree on what

reasons count as public for the purpose of public justification, a political decision based on any of those reasons can be legitimately implemented even
if some people oppose it (e.g. because they interpret or weigh the underlying
reasons in different ways from those who endorse the decision). Even though
Lister does not frame his analysis in terms of the tripartite distinction that we
adopt in this chapter, and does not clearly distinguish between reasons and
evaluative standards, his account shares with the accessibility conception of
public reason both the view that we can appeal to shared criteria to establish
what reasons should and should not be allowed into the process of public justification and the idea that public justification can be inconclusive.

We would also like to stress that it is important for participants in public reasoning under accessibility to consider *all* the shared political values potentially
involved in the justification for a political decision. As pointed out by Quong,
if public justification fails to consider some of the political values involved in a
policy decision, that may result in an unreasonable balance of political values.
This kind of balance, i.e., can be the consequence not only of an undue prioritization of certain political values over others (once all the values involved in
the balancing have been taken into account) but also of a total neglect of certain
values which, therefore, are not even included in the balancing process. One
way of including such values in an actual process of public justification is to
engage in counterfactual or hypothetical reasoning (e.g. 'what if one objected
to this policy by arguing that it fails to take into account shared political value
x?'). However, the decision-making framework that we develop in Chapter 7
will aim to institutionalize this process via various forms of community-based
forums, consultation procedures, and deliberative settings in the design of
healthy eating efforts. These forums would aim to ensure that key political
values relevant to the formulation and implementation of healthy eating efforts
are not neglected during the process of public justification, e.g. by empowering
local communities to call public attention to those values that are particularly
important to them, and which may otherwise be overlooked in the design of
healthy eating efforts.

But let's return to the inconclusiveness of public reason, which is widely
acknowledged and accepted by defenders of consensus accounts of public
reason (Cross and Besch 2019), and which implies that conflicting accessible reasons do not act as defeaters but simply express different political
conceptions of justice, which may sometimes support different (and even
conflicting) policies. Rawls (2005b, p. 451) himself argues that political liberalism 'does not try to fix public reason once and for all in the form of one

favoured political conception of justice' and allows instead 'a family of political conceptions of justice' (p. 450). Based on this view, therefore, it can be argued that accessible reasons cannot act as defeaters against certain laws, policies, and programmes (including healthy eating efforts), when the latter are grounded in accessible reasons that reflect a reasonable balance of political values.[3]

It could be observed, of course, that there is no intrinsic connection between accessibility, as a conception of the structure of public reason, and the idea that laws whose underlying accessible reasons reflect a reasonable balance of political values cannot be defeated by the mere fact that other members of the public endorse other accessible reasons reflecting a different reasonable balance of political values. Indeed one could imagine a different conception of accessibility in which the accessible reasons of some members of the public, like intelligible reasons under the intelligibility conception, do count as defeaters against laws grounded in different accessible reasons. Under that conception, as under intelligibility, it is likely that many healthy eating efforts would indeed be defeated by the accessible reasons of those citizens who oppose such efforts (and their underlying accessible reasons). But that would the facto imply reverting from an accessibility to a shareability conception of public reason, in which all citizens are expected to endorse not only the evaluative standards that underlie a reason used to justify a policy but also the reason itself, including the specific balance of political values reflected by that reason. And we have already shown that shareability does not allow much scope for healthy eating efforts.

We would like to conclude our analysis in this chapter with a further consideration. We previously acknowledged that there might be objections to healthy eating efforts unrelated to public reason and public justification. Those objections, we saw, might concern the effectiveness and efficiency of such efforts, their excessively coercive and intrusive nature, and the harm they may cause. It now seems, however, that those concerns can be reconceptualized (at least in some cases) within the framework of public justification and public reason, and of accessibility more specifically. Assessing the effectiveness or efficiency of a policy, e.g., requires appealing to shared epistemic evaluative standards (e.g. widely endorsed methods of economic analysis and social science). Likewise, establishing whether a healthy eating

---

[3] Accessible reasons could, of course, act as defeaters against laws grounded in an *unreasonable* balance of political values.

effort is excessively coercive and intrusive involves assessing whether it overly interferes with people's individual rights and liberties, which are shared moral evaluative standards. Similarly, it can be assumed that people in liberal societies share a general conception of harm, which also constitutes a moral evaluative standard based on which the harmfulness of healthy eating efforts can be assessed (e.g. Cohen 2010, pp. 272–77). While these are certainly complex issues, the key point is that they can be reconceptualized within the framework of public reason and public justification that we have examined in this chapter. By appealing to shared epistemic and moral evaluative standards, i.e., we can assess many of the implications of healthy eating efforts in diverse societies.

5.4. From direct to indirect public reason

Is public reason consistent with healthy eating efforts? In this chapter we addressed this question by examining the three main conceptions of the structure of public reason that can be found in the literature: accessibility, shareability, and intelligibility. We argued that under both the 'intelligibility' conception and the 'shareability' conception the majority of healthy eating efforts would not be publicly justified. More specifically, under the intelligibility conception any intelligible reasons could defeat such efforts, whereas under the shareability conception there would be very few (if any) reasons that all members of the public can affirm as their own and, consequently, very few (if any) publicly justified healthy eating efforts. We therefore concluded that healthy eating efforts are compatible with public reason only if one endorses an 'accessibility' conception. According to this conception, political rules are publicly justified if they are based on reasons grounded in shared epistemic and moral evaluative standards, as long as such reasons reflect a reasonable balance of political values and do not overly prioritize or neglect any of these values. This implies that at least some healthy eating efforts that are not justified by appealing to shared reasons—e.g. policies and interventions that secure health gains by imposing sacrifices that conflict with many people's values and beliefs—can still be publicly justified by appealing to accessible reasons, as long as such reasons reflect a reasonable balance of political values.

We believe that our argument has important implications for healthy eating efforts and beyond. Public reason scholars, and especially critics of public reason, should more often recognize the difference between fully endorsing a reason for a policy, in the spirit of shareability, and seeing that reason as providing a reasonable balance of political values that they share. (And we will see in the next chapter that this scenario is complicated once we pay more attention to the complex interrelationship between different types of evaluative standards, i.e. factual, metaphysical, epistemic, and moral.)

Acknowledging this difference can be important not only to help avoid the risk of policy inaction, a risk that we saw is associated especially with the intelligibility and shareability conceptions of public reason. It can also help citizens overcome the risk of political polarization that increasingly characterizes liberal democracies. And it is interesting to note that in an attempt to put forward a recipe for social trust and cooperation to overcome polarization, and in response to the previously mentioned 'anarchy objection' (Vallier 2019, p. 114), in one of his most recent works Vallier argues that 'members of the public are not concerned with living according to their evaluative standards alone, since they also value cooperating with others. And members of the public may also include among their evaluative standards the need to get along and even be reconciled to others' (p. 115). Vallier's statement is a (perhaps unintentional) recognition that only by stressing what we share can we hope to overcome deep divisions within society. Both intelligibility and shareability, in different ways, put emphasis instead on what we do *not* share: intelligibility highlights those reasons and evaluative standards that are related to individuals' comprehensive doctrines; shareability emphasizes instead reasons that we allegedly share with all the other members of our political community but which, we have seen, do not actually exist.

It may still be difficult, though, to ensure that members of the public (as opposed to professional philosophers) fully grasp and embrace the distinction between different models of public reason. When healthy eating efforts are debated, e.g. at the community level, some participants may dominate and polarize the discussion by emphasizing sources of division rather than what participants share. However, it should be noted that this is an issue only if one believes that the constraints of public reason apply to all citizens, which is what Rawls and other defenders of a direct model of public reason argue. This model of public reason, which entails a *direct* exclusion of non-public reasons from public deliberation, is potentially very exclusive and has indeed been criticized for undermining the integrity of religious citizens (who are asked to set aside their religious beliefs during public deliberation) and for being unfair towards them (compared to non-religious citizens) (Vallier 2014; Wolterstorff 1997).

However, there is an alternative model of public reason, the *indirect* one, which imposes the constraints of public reason only upon public officials (judges, elected politicians, public health officers, etc.) and institutions but not upon ordinary citizens (Bonotti 2017, pp. 124–51; Vallier 2014, pp. 50–51). More specifically,

> an indirect method allows citizens to forgo explicit attempts in political de-
> liberation and action to bar excluded reasons from playing a justificatory
> role. The indirect approach focuses instead on regulating *the behavior of
> politicians and the structure of political institutions* to ensure that excluded
> reasons do not generate publicly unjustified law. (Vallier 2014, p. 51, em-
> phasis added)

This model, which we prefer, allows a much more inclusive debate amongst ordinary citizens concerning healthy eating efforts. And even though it may from time to time lead to polarized debates, e.g. when such efforts are discussed at the community level, it is the task of public officials, and especially policymakers, to formulate accessible public reason in support of healthy eating efforts which take into account the public and non-public reasons emerging from debates amongst citizens. How to ensure that there is an institutional link between policymakers and citizen forums is an issue to which we will return in Chapter 7, where we defend the need for mechanisms of deliberation and consultation in the design of healthy eating efforts.

6

Unreasonable Healthy Eating Efforts

6.1. Introduction

In the previous chapter we argued that only the accessibility conception of public reason is consistent with healthy eating efforts. Accessible reasons are those grounded in evaluative standards that are shared at some level of idealization amongst the members of a political community despite their different conceptions of the good. We argued that the accessibility conception of public reason is preferable to shareability and intelligibility because neither of these alternative conceptions would allow (almost) any healthy eating efforts. The former is too demanding (given the fact of reasonable pluralism, there are no shared reasons in diverse societies), the latter is too permissive (given the fact of reasonable pluralism, there are too many intelligible reasons in diverse societies, and such reasons could be used by individual citizens to defeat most if not all healthy eating efforts). The accessibility conception of public reason therefore seems to strike the right balance between demandingness and permissiveness.

In this chapter we intend to show that the accessibility conception of public reason provides a useful conceptual and normative framework for critically assessing existing and proposed healthy eating efforts in liberal democracies. In other words, we want to develop a critical tool for establishing when healthy eating efforts are unreasonable, i.e. publicly unjustified and therefore illegitimate. In the literature on political liberalism, the term 'unreasonable' is often used to refer to individuals or doctrines that reject liberal democratic values and institutions, and reject 'the equal provision of basic rights and opportunities across society' (Badano and Nuti 2018, p. 150; see also Badano and Nuti 2020; Clayton and Stevens 2014). Or, to be more specific, drawing on Rawls's on terminology, 'unreasonable' citizens (and doctrines) are those that fail to comply with the two demands of reasonableness, i.e. '[being] ready to propose principles and standards as fair terms of cooperation and to abide by them willingly, given the assurance that others will likewise do so' (Rawls 2005a, p. 49),

Healthy Eating Policy and Political Philosophy. Anne Barnhill and Matteo Bonotti, Oxford University Press. © Oxford University Press 2022. DOI: 10.1093/oso/9780190937881.003.0007

and '[being willing] to recognize the burdens of judgment and to accept their consequences for the use of public reason in directing the legitimate exercise of political power in a constitutional regime' (Rawls 2005a, p. 54). While drawing on this definition of unreasonableness, here we understand the term 'unreasonable' more broadly, as involving the illegitimate exercise of political power based on non-public reasons grounded in controversial comprehensive doctrines (Rawls 2005a, p. 138), even if this does not pose a threat to liberal democratic values and institutions, or infringe upon some citizens' rights and opportunities. However, we intend to move beyond the well-rehearsed but rather generic argument that political power, and specifically in our case its exercise via healthy eating efforts, is illegitimate when grounded in controversial ethical, philosophical, or religious doctrines. Instead, we intend to unpack the concept of 'evaluative standards', which is central to the accessibility conception of public reason, and show that (a) there are different categories of evaluative standards relevant to accessibility and (b) for each category we can identify ways in which healthy eating efforts and objections to them can be unreasonable, i.e. not compliant with the accessibility view of public reason.

We draw more specifically on Badano and Bonotti's (2020) and Vallier's (2016) recent work in order to develop a categorization of evaluative standards that will allow us to explain in what sense different types of healthy eating efforts are unreasonable. Evaluative standards can be both 'prescriptive and descriptive' (Vallier 2016, p. 607). Descriptive evaluative standards, we argue, can be both *factual* and *metaphysical*, and prescriptive evaluative standards can be both *epistemic* and *moral*. We will first introduce each of these categories, and then examine them in relation to healthy eating efforts (see Table 6.1).

6.2. Categorizing evaluating standards

6.2.1. Prescriptive epistemic evaluative standards

Let's start by considering *prescriptive epistemic evaluative standards*. These include epistemic rules employed for the collection of factual evidence and for drawing inferences. They correspond to what Rawls (2005a, p. 223) calls 'guidelines of inquiry', without which 'substantive principles cannot be applied'. The scientific method also constitutes a set of prescriptive epistemic

Table 6.1 Types of Evaluative Standards and Examples

Type of evaluative standard	Examples of shared standards	Examples of non-shared standards	Examples from debates about healthy eating efforts
Prescriptive epistemic evaluative standards	Standards of scientific inquiry	'Bad' science Pseudo-science	Using the BMI to assert facts about overweight and obesity
Descriptive factual evaluative standards (the kind of facts that are the subject of study in the natural and social sciences)	Factual claims from majority science Factual claims from minority science	Factual claims from 'bad' science, pseudo-science, or incomplete/ selective science E.g. 'Taking hydroxychloroquine to treat COVID-19 is safe and effective'	Claiming that in the US, sugary drinks are consumed in quantities that pose health risks—*based on shared evaluative standards and therefore reasonable* Claiming that dietary patterns do not have any significant relationship with health—*based on unshared evaluative standards (bad science) and therefore unreasonable* Healthy eating efforts that fail to take into account relevant facts concerning their social, psychological, and economic effects—*incomplete scientific evidence and failure to consider the 'strains of commitment', therefore unreasonable* Industry actors with self-interested/ sectarian agendas drawing on scientific research in ways that downplay limitations of and disagreements in the empirical evidence available—*selective/ incomplete/self-interested use of scientific evidence, therefore unreasonable*

Descriptive metaphysical evaluative standards (metaphysical beliefs, broadly construed)	Commonsense metaphysical beliefs E.g. objects persist over time	Metaphysical beliefs rooted in non-shared religious, supernatural or folk belief systems E.g. the belief that human foetuses have souls	Food taboos Beliefs about the natural that are grounded in moral, aesthetic, or other ideational reasons—*based on non-shared metaphysical evaluative standards and therefore unreasonable*
Prescriptive moral evaluative standards	Shared political values E.g. basic liberties and rights, equality of opportunity, the common good	Values rooted in religious doctrines E.g. Catholic or Islamic religious principles	Designing healthy eating efforts to maximize public health benefits without paying attention to whether the efforts disproportionately burden certain groups—*failure to consider the 'strains of commitment', therefore unreasonable* Failing to consider/assigning insufficient importance to racial or gender inequality when designing healthy eating efforts—*unreasonable balance of political values* Assuming that consumption of an unhealthy food has no value—*unreasonable balance of political values* Assigning insufficient or excessive importance to individual freedom and consumer choice—*unreasonable balance of political values*

evaluative standards which are widely shared, both amongst scientists and, at least in principle, amongst the general public in liberal democracies (Badano and Bonotti 2020).

Here a clarification is required. Science (including the science which lies at the basis of much healthy eating policy) involves specific evaluative standards that most people do not know or understand. However, it can be argued that these standards are still shared in the relevant sense. There are different ways of defending this claim. One is by saying that the general public *in principle* shares these standards, i.e. that if members of the public devoted sufficient time and energy to understanding them, they would be able to understand them, and would accept them as valid. This way of arguing that scientific evaluative standards are shared by the public involves only a moderate level of idealization, i.e. the view that citizens with normal human capacities may be able to passively understand (rather than actively develop) key scientific methods and conclusions (Badano and Bonotti 2020).[1] Another way of arguing that scientific evaluative standards are shared by the public is this: if the public accepts science and its validity in general (an assumption that we think can be safely made about many societies), then it implicitly accepts the more specific methods and epistemic standards of science. However, this second option may be problematic because it is more dependent on an empirical claim that could be disproved. Disputes concerning vaccinations and public health interventions during the COVID-19 pandemic in the US, e.g., showed that perhaps a not insignificant percentage of the public in that country may not accept science and its validity in general. Therefore a degree of idealization seems necessary if we want to avoid the problems that a more populist (i.e. less idealized) account of public reason might result in.

Even if we accept that people in liberal democracies normally share prescriptive epistemic evaluative standards, however, we should also acknowledge that they may employ them in different ways and thus reach different conclusions. For example, scientists may follow the same (widely shared) scientific methods and still reach different scientific conclusions, something that is perhaps more likely to happen in the social than in the natural sciences,

---

[1] At this point one might still object that a person with normal human capacities might also understand and accept religion and its evaluative standards. However, there is a clear asymmetry between religion and science: '[w]hile there are people who believe that only science is a source of truth, and people who believe that both science and religion are sources of truth, almost no one believes that only religion constitutes a source of truth' (Badano and Bonotti 2020, p. 63).

given their subject of study. Here we understand scientific methods in a very broad sense, since we acknowledge that scientists may disagree not only with regard to their conclusions but also with regard to the specific methods they employ in their everyday research, and that testing methods (as well as conclusions) via trial and error, allowing for a plurality of perspectives, is in itself a key aspect of scientific inquiry.

When scientists draw on broadly shared methods and still disagree in their conclusions, such conclusions can still provide grounds for accessible reasons. However, for this to be the case, no 'gross epistemic error' (Vallier 2014, p. 106) must have been made by the relevant scientists in their reasoning process and in their use of scientific methods and other shared epistemic evaluative standards. A 'gross epistemic error' may be made, e.g., when

A fails to consider a counterexample to a generalisation her reason R_A rests on, or if R_A mistakes a sufficient for a necessary condition, or if she forgets or gives little weight to an important value consideration when the values relevant to a law are balanced against one another. (Badano and Bonotti 2020, p. 38)

If no gross epistemic error is made, and different conclusions are reached simply due to the burdens of judgement that inevitably affect any human inquiry, then both the prescriptive epistemic evaluative standards employed in scientific inquiry and the factual claims resulting from their use are shared, and therefore are a source of accessible public reasons.

All of this implies that disagreement amongst scientists is a healthy aspect of accessible public reasoning, rather than a burden to it. Yet we should also note that sometimes, perhaps often, the scientific community is not evenly divided. That is, there might be a majority view which most researchers embrace, and one or more minority views endorsed by a smaller section of the scientific community. Crucially, this may not necessarily be due to any gross epistemic errors made in the use of scientific methods. It is therefore a genuine and legitimate disagreement, and minority views can legitimately count as accessible public reasons.

However, we believe that the fact that some views are in the minority should be taken into account somehow during the process of public justification. We will return to this point later in the chapter, when discussing healthy eating efforts more specifically, as this type of uneven disagreement is especially relevant to scientific debates on healthy eating. For now, based on this consideration, it is useful to distinguish between different types of 'good' and 'bad' scientific positions.

First, there is what we may call *majority science*, science that uses shared evaluative standards without making any gross epistemic errors and reaches conclusions endorsed by the majority in the scientific community. Second, there is *minority science*, i.e. science that employs shared evaluative standards without making any gross epistemic errors but reaches conclusions endorsed by only a minority within the scientific community. It is important to note that majority and minority positions are not crystallized. Sometimes there can be waves of consensus, so that what constitutes a majority position at one time becomes a minority position later on, and vice versa (Shwed and Bearman 2010). Third, there is *bad science*. This is science that draws on shared scientific evaluative standards but, by making gross epistemic errors, produces wrong conclusions, e.g. climate science denial. Finally, there is what we might call *pseudo-science*. This constitutes a distinctive epistemic community, different from the previous three. Its members may not be making any gross epistemic errors (though sometimes they do); they simply employ different evaluative standards from those embraced by the other three groups. For example, some vaccine hesitancy and opposition to approved vaccines is rooted in pseudo-science, which relies on prescriptive epistemic evaluative standards that are not those of science (Hornsey et al. 2018). For another example of pseudo-science, consider Trump's statement, during the COVID-19 pandemic, that '[t]aking hydroxychloroquine to treat COVID-19 is safe and effective' (Dale 2020; Paz 2020), a claim he continued to make even after being challenged by the scientific community (Carvalho 2020). In making this claim, Trump relied on a French study (Gautret 2020) that was later judged scientifically flawed (Wong 2020) and could be considered an example of bad science. What rendered Trump's statement an instance of pseudo-science, however, was the fact that, in making it, he appealed to his own personal beliefs as if these were on a par with scientific evidence. When Anthony Fauci, director of the US National Institute of Allergy and Infectious Diseases, denied that the drug hydroxychloroquine is effective at preventing COVID-19, Trump rebutted, '[i]t may work, it may not work. I feel good about it. That's all it is, it's just a feeling, you know, right, smart guy' (World News Tonight 2020). But *feelings* are not sources of valid scientific knowledge. Appealing to them, therefore, can produce only pseudo-scientific findings.[2]

---

[2] For an analysis of these issues, see Bonotti and Zech (2021, Chap. 4).

6.2.2. *Descriptive factual evaluative standards*

Descriptive factual evaluative standards include the kinds of facts that are the subject of study in the natural and social sciences. The sense in which these facts are 'evaluative standards' is that we use them to assess reasons. If a reason offered for a policy refers to facts that are not true, then that reason is not accessible.

These factual evaluative standards include, for example, the fact that the earth is round, that WWII ended in 1945, or that China is the most populous country in the world. It is important to stress that factual standards, even when more sophisticated and complex than the ones we have just mentioned, are not just the prerogative of natural and social scientists. Indeed, we saw earlier, Rawls (2005a, p. 224, emphasis added) himself argues that public reason also includes 'presently accepted general beliefs and forms of reasoning *found in common sense*'. There is a difference in degree, but not in kind, between the kind of knowledge that natural and social scientists can produce and that which lay persons can produce and understand: '[s]cience is not a substitute for common sense, but an extension [although more complex and sophisticated] of it' (Quine 1957, p. 2). Factual standards can be shared (like the ones mentioned earlier) or unshared (e.g. the view that the earth is flat). Only the former can provide the grounds for accessible reasons.

Reasons may be based on factual standards that are not widely known amongst the general public (e.g. compared to facts such as that the earth is round) but are still the result of scientific norms/scientific consensus and thus are 'in principle' shared. As in the case of prescriptive epistemic evaluative standards, what matters is that people accept science generally, or that they could in principle passively understand the same facts if they dedicated a sufficient amount of time and energy to this endeavour. Furthermore, since in most liberal democracies the vast majority of citizens consider science a reliable source for establishing factual truths, whatever facts science discovers can be considered shared by the members of the general public even if the latter do not understand in any detail what they involve.

6.2.3. *Descriptive metaphysical evaluative standards*

Next, let's consider what we call *descriptive metaphysical evaluative standards*. These include metaphysical beliefs such as religious beliefs or beliefs related to supernatural or folk worldviews, the truth of which cannot be established via scientific enquiry. One example is Catholics' view 'that God imbues foetuses with souls at conception, or more accurately, that in the act of the creation of a human person, God creates a being with both substantial form (the soul) and matter' (Vallier 2016, p. 608). This view, along with many other religious beliefs and beliefs related to supernatural worldviews, are likely to be unshared in most societies. But many basic metaphysical beliefs may be shared in a society, and may be part of its public political culture. These may include, e.g., beliefs about the identity of persons or the persistence of objects over time.

6.2.4. *Prescriptive moral evaluative standards*

Finally, there are what we call *prescriptive moral evaluative standards*. These may be grounded, e.g., in religious doctrines or specific ethical worldviews, and in such cases they are generally controversial. But they may also be grounded in what Rawls calls a political conception of justice, and in this case they provide a shared moral vocabulary rooted in the public political culture of a liberal democratic society. For example, while Islamic, Catholic, or Buddhist prescriptive moral evaluative standards are definitely unshared in liberal democracies, certain political values are widely shared (at some level of idealization) and constitute grounds for accessible public reasons.

According to Rawls (2005a, p. 291), shared political values include basic liberties such as 'freedom of thought and liberty of conscience; the political liberties and freedom of association, as well as the freedoms specified by the liberty and integrity of the person; and finally, the rights and liberties covered by the rule of law'. They also comprise 'the right to hold and to have the exclusive use of personal property' (p. 298), 'equality of opportunity', and 'values of the common good' (p. 224), which include promoting public health, since public health institutions help 'to reproduce political society over time' (Rawls 2005b, pp. 456–57). Finally, political values also include 'the various necessary conditions for all these values' (Rawls 2005a, p. 224). These comprise a 'social minimum' (Rawls 2005a, p. 228), i.e. a set of goods that helps people to fulfil their basic needs and thus protects them from such conditions as hunger or disease (Kaufman 2018, pp. 223–24), and health is arguably one such good.[3]

---

[3] See also Daniels (2008).

We would like to emphasize that appealing to shared political values can also help us condemn various forms of structural injustice that pervade contemporary liberal democracies. While Rawls' theory of justice has been criticized for overlooking structural injustice (e.g. Powers and Faden 2019), given its overemphasis on basic rights and liberties as well as redistribution of resources, we think that his account of public reason can offer a critical lens on structural injustice, especially since it allows 'a *family* of political conceptions of justice, and not. . . a single one' (Rawls 2005b, p. 450, emphasis added). These political conceptions of justice arguably include those on which justice requires the absence of structural injustice. Thus, even if Rawls' own theory of justice was silent on structural injustice, his conception of public reason allows conceptions of justice that speak to structural justice. One might also argue that structural injustice contributes to undermining the self-respect of members of oppressed and vulnerable groups, and self-respect is also a shared political value in liberal democracies, i.e. one that all reasonable citizens ought to desire for each and every member of the political community. As Rawls (1999, p. 386) points out, self-respect involves

> a person's sense of his own value, his secure conviction that his conception of his good, his plan of life, is worth carrying out . . . [as well as] a confidence in one's ability, so far as it is within one's power, to fulfill one's intentions.

Finally, structural injustice also creates fertile ground for what Rawls calls the 'strains of commitment' (p. 153), which we will discuss shortly. In addition, a case can be made that Rawlsian justice *requires* the absence of structural injustice, even though Rawls himself did not make that link. For example, structural injustice could reasonably be considered a threat to (fair) equality of opportunity, on some reasonable conceptions of equality of opportunity (cf. Jugov and Ypi 2019).

It is important to stress that while sharing these political values, members of liberal societies may endorse different interpretations of them. In the case of basic rights and liberties, diversity of interpretations may seem to be less significant than for other shared political values. Rawls (2005a, p. 86) himself states that 'it is much easier to gain agreement about what the basic rights and liberties should be, not in every detail of course, but about the main outline'. Yet, disagreement may still be present. For example, when it comes to freedom of speech, some citizens may believe that this involves absolute freedom from state interference, whereas others may believe that the correct understanding of free speech is *equal freedom of speech for all*, which may justify regulating speech that creates or reinforces power asymmetries amongst citizens (e.g. hate speech, pornography, and commercial speech), or *positive freedom* that requires some degree of state support for (some) citizens' speech. In the case of other political values, such as equality of opportunity or the common good, disagreement may be even more significant. For example, citizens may disagree as to whether equality of opportunity should be formal or 'fair' (Rawls 1999), or as to whether the general good is mainly driven by economic growth or public health. To give another example, citizens may disagree about the specific remedies for structural racism and the forms of racial equity that are required by justice (e.g. in the US context, does justice require reparations for slavery, and of what form?). The accessibility conception of public reason allows these kinds of disagreements. Accessibility also allows disagreement between different ways of balancing shared political values, as in Quong's (2011, p. 205) example of Tony and Sara discussed in the previous chapter.

6.3. Examples of evaluative standards in debates about healthy eating efforts

Having briefly illustrated the four categories of evaluative standards central to accessibility, we will now explain their relevance to healthy eating efforts. We will discuss some examples in which shared evaluative standards, and controversial evaluative standards, underlie healthy eating efforts or underlie objections to healthy eating efforts.

6.3.1. Examples of descriptive factual evaluative standards and prescriptive epistemic evaluative standards in healthy eating policy debates

First of all, we would like to discuss descriptive factual evaluative standards and prescriptive epistemic evaluative standards. We discuss them together because they are closely related: epistemic evaluative standards are employed to reach conclusions about natural and social facts. When it comes to healthy eating efforts, and the reasons invoked to justify them, factual evaluative standards may include facts concerning health, illness, and food, and the relationship between them. What kind of issues may arise here?

First, healthy eating efforts could be justified by appealing to reasons grounded in controversial factual claims about the connection between eating and health (or lack thereof). For example, there is significant empirical uncertainty or disagreement surrounding the ways in which childhood obesity is measured and the effectiveness of public health interventions to target obesity (Voigt et al. 2014). Some critics of healthy eating efforts highlight these issues. This is one of those cases where, as shown in the previous section, scientists may share the same evaluative standards but reach different conclusions, with some being in the majority and others in the minority. Other examples of uncertainty and disagreement include the health effects of certain kinds of consumption, and the optimal levels of consumption for health—e.g. disagreement about the optimal level of sodium consumption to reduce disease and mortality (Kolata 2013; The Nutrition Source 2013) and disagreement about whether saturated fat intake contributes to cardiovascular disease and whether reducing such intake has health benefits (Svendsen et al. 2017). More generally, on many issues concerning the health effects of food, there are views that are endorsed by the majority in the scientific community, and views that are in the minority, even though the latter are not the result of gross epistemic errors.

Minority views can have a role in the public justification of healthy eating efforts since they can still be sources of accessible reasons. However, to require minority scientific views to always have a hearing may be time-consuming and unnecessary. For example, if the majority of scientists argue that saturated fats are bad for health, should policymakers and the general public have to listen to those who argue otherwise? Arguably, when it comes to public justification, we cannot simply consider whether the reasons for a policy are accessible or not. We also need to consider the relative weight that different views have within the scientific community. Since it is a generally endorsed belief that policymaking should be effective and efficient, investing too much time in listening to all positions, and including all those views that are in the minority, may not contribute to that goal. (This may be especially the case when governments face public health emergencies, e.g. the COVID-19 pandemic.)

How, then, could minority views be dealt with during the process of public justification? Expert committees could regularly assess the full set of scientific evidence (e.g. evidence about the health effects of sodium consumption), give both minority and majority views a hearing, and reach conclusions meant to guide policymaking. Then, in its normal operations, a public health agency could perhaps consider only the conclusions reached by expert bodies when publicly justifying a healthy eating policy, given the aforementioned importance of effectiveness and efficiency in policymaking.

Alternatively, if the process of public justification is being carried out, say, as part of a deliberative forum discussing one or more healthy eating efforts, perhaps a moderator/facilitator should highlight the status (i.e. minority or majority) of the views discussed before or during the deliberative process, so that participants are aware of this. A difficult question is whether, when policymaking happens at the community level and is community-driven (e.g. a town designs healthy eating efforts for itself, rather than efforts being designed at the state or province level), it could be acceptable for the community to endorse a policy based on minority science. In other words, does the minority status of certain scientific positions always *entail* that they should not ground public health efforts? Or should citizens, when they are involved in the design of healthy eating efforts at various levels, decide which scientific views those efforts should be based on? One position on this issue may be that if citizens decide to proceed with a policy recommendation based on minority scientific views, then that should be considered publicly justified and democratically legitimate (even though not always epistemically optimal), so long as citizens were made aware of the status of different views within the scientific community, i.e. whether they are majority or minority views. A divergent position on this issue may be that citizens, even when making decisions only for themselves (i.e. a policy for their town), should generally have to hew to majority science, given that efforts based on minority science are less likely to be effective, and thus less likely to promote the broadly shared political values that ultimately justify them.

Let's now consider some more specific examples of healthy eating efforts that fail to be grounded in shared factual evaluative standards and/or prescriptive epistemic evaluative standards.

6.3.1.1. Bad science and healthy eating efforts

Some might try to justify or criticize healthy eating efforts by engaging in what is de facto bad science, making gross epistemic errors while drawing on shared epistemic evaluative standards. For example, suppose that someone asserted that dietary patterns do not have any significant relationship with health, and therefore promoting healthier dietary patterns should not be the focus of any public health efforts. The claim that dietary patterns do not have any significant relationship with health is controversial, since there is broad agreement regarding the link between dietary patterns and health risks. In other words, this claim is controversial in a way that is different from the controversy that characterizes the previously examined claim that minimizing saturated fat consumption is optimal for health. In that case, there is a legitimate disagreement amongst scientists about a specific claim, whereas there is not the same kind of disagreement about the broad claim that dietary patterns are linked to health. This is not to say that the relationship between dietary patterns and health is in all respects clear and uncontroversial amongst scientists; it is not.

6.3.1.2. Disagreement and body mass index

Let's now consider a case of genuine disagreement. There is uncertainty and disagreement surrounding the use of the body mass index (BMI) to measure obesity. The BMI is a function of body mass and height (body mass in kilograms/height in m^2), and overweight and obesity are standardly measured using the BMI (overweight is a BMI of 25 or greater, and obesity is a BMI greater than 30). A number of scholars have indeed criticized the use of the BMI as a measure of overweight and obesity, especially with regard to individuals who are located at the lower end of the overweight spectrum. Critics have especially highlighted the lack of precision that characterizes the BMI which, e.g., does not take into account the distribution and position of fat within the body, especially in relation to other aspects of body mass such as muscles and bones (Voigt et al. 2014). This results in some people being considered overweight even though they may have a relatively low level of body fat. There is also some evidence that people who are overweight (but not obese) based on BMI assessment have lower mortality than normal-weight people, though there is also evidence that people who are overweight at some point during adulthood have higher mortality (Flegal et al. 2013; Wang et al. 2016). Thus, one could argue that for the purposes of public health efforts, the BMI is an imperfect way of characterizing body state, because it does not capture what matters most to health. This seems to be another case where scientists agreeing on shared epistemic evaluative standards reach different conclusions.

But the problem here seems to be different from the one characterizing cases of mere disagreement amongst scientists. In this case, some might argue that the BMI is such a poor construct that we cannot justify continuing to use it, or to use data based on it. Especially if there are other measures (e.g. measuring body fat) that would be superior to the BMI in the crucial respect (i.e. they would measure a feature of bodies that is more reliably connected to health), how could continued use of the BMI be justifiable? Yet this conclusion may be too hurried. Suppose that the BMI, while admittedly very imperfect, is nonetheless a more practicable measure: the BMI of individuals can be more easily measured by healthcare providers, health researchers, and those implementing and evaluating healthy eating interventions, as compared to alternative measures. Thus, despite the limitations of the BMI, given the difficulty in devising and employing other types of measurement, it is conceivable that the BMI could be the best practical tool we can use to characterize body state for the purpose of gathering data about weight and health.

This example tells us something more general about public reason. Perhaps appealing to slightly controversial standards is acceptable in view of complex real-world circumstances, and of the practical and financial limits within which public policy often must operate.

6.3.1.3. Nutritionism

Let's consider another example of how healthy eating efforts could be rooted in controversial factual claims. According to some critics, healthy eating efforts are rooted in *nutritionism*, an ideology that involves controversial factual claims concerning food and health. Scrinis (2008, p. 41), e.g., understands nutritionism as involving 'food level reductionism', i.e. a view in which 'individual foods either tend to be fetishized as "super foods" or vilified, usually on the basis of their underlying nutrient composition', leading to a 'decontextualization of single foods out of the contexts in which they are usually consumed'. According to Scrinis (2013, Chap. 5), nutritionism has been central to many healthy eating efforts, e.g. government nutrition education campaigns such as the Low-Fat, Low-Calorie, and Low-Carb ones. Nutritionism, as described by Scrinis, neglects the importance of *whole diets* in promoting health and singles out individual foods as intrinsically good or bad for health. For example, the American Dietetic Association (Nitzke et al. 2007, p. 1226) (now renamed Academy of Nutrition and Dietetics (AND)) has argued that there are no intrinsically 'good' or 'bad' foods, and that 'the total diet approach, with its emphasis on long-term eating habits and a contextual approach to food judgments . . . provides more useful information to guide long-term food choices'.

Thus the criticism is that some healthy eating efforts are rooted in, and promote, a model of healthy eating (on which some foods are intrinsically bad) that is less accurate and useful than an alternative approach that focuses on whole diets. But arguably, healthy eating efforts are not typically grounded in the decontextualization of foods outside the context of a whole diet, and are not based in the belief that *any* amount of foods high in fat, sugar, or salt is bad for health. For example, the US dietary guidelines include the following recommendation, which focuses on the overall dietary pattern: '[l]imit calories from added sugars and saturated fats and reduce sodium intake. Consume an eating pattern low in added sugars, saturated fats, and sodium. Cut back on foods and beverages higher in these components to amounts that fit within healthy eating patterns' (US Department of Health and Human Services and US Department of Agriculture 2015).

Some healthy eating efforts do focus on specific foods; e.g. numerous efforts and policies aim to reduce consumption of sugary drinks. Arguably, though, those policies are not based in the view that *any* amount of sugary drink consumption is intrinsically bad, but rather are rooted in empirical evidence that sugary drinks are *in fact* consumed at levels that pose health risks. For example, sugary drinks are a primary source of added sugar in the US diet, and empirical evidence links sugary drink consumption with caloric consumption, weight gain, obesity, diabetes, and hypertension, amongst other health conditions (Lynch and Bassler 2014). Similarly, other healthy eating recommendations and efforts, such as those promoting greater consumption of fruits and vegetables, are based on empirical evidence showing that these foods are generally under-consumed and higher consumption would reduce the risk of diet-related illness (Afshin et al. 2019). Thus, one aspect of the ideology of nutritionism—the decontextualization of foods outside the context of a whole diet, and the belief that *any* amount of certain foods is bad for health—does not seem generally to characterize healthy eating efforts.

However, nutritionism also involves another dimension, i.e. the view that we should 'think about foods in terms of their nutrient composition ... make the connection between particular nutrients and bodily health ... and ... construct "nutritionally balanced" diets on this basis' (Scrinis 2008, p. 39). This aspect of nutritionism, it should be noted, is not controversial *tout court*. The view that an excess of certain nutrients, such as sodium, is bad for health is uncontroversial, both amongst the scientific community and the general public, as is the view that eating too much food high in these nutrients (e.g. packaged and processed food that is high in sodium) is bad for health. Furthermore, it is undisputable that some micronutrient deficiencies (e.g. iron, vitamin A, vitamin D, folic acid, and calcium) have negative effects on people's health, and focusing on specific nutrients can be useful for tackling these problems from a scientific perspective (Jacobs and Tapsell 2007, p. 447). However, nutritionism is considered problematic by some in its assumptions that (a) only specific nutrients count and (b) we can build a healthy diet (or even a 'perfect' diet) from the ground up by combining the 'right' nutrients, what Scrinis (2008) refers to as 'nutritional reductionism'. According to this criticism, nutritionism neglects the importance that whole foods play in people's diet, above and beyond the sum of their constituent nutrients. In other words, *foods qua whole foods* have an added value that is not reducible to the mere sum of their nutrients.[4] Thus, if healthy eating efforts were rooted in the factual claim that optimal diets can be built from the ground up by combining the right nutrients, then they would be criticizable from this perspective.

The debate on nutritionism therefore reveals, once again, the presence of disagreement about factual claims concerning the relationship between eating and health (what we are referring to as 'descriptive factual evaluative standards'). And this disagreement may also concern the methodological approach to the development of healthy eating efforts. For example, as an alternative to a nutritionist approach, which aims to build an ideal healthy diet from the bottom up, others have defended approaches that appeal to historical practices and evidence in order to provide people with healthy eating guidelines (e.g. Piscopo 2009; Trichopolus et al. 2000).

We have already stressed, however, that the presence of this kind of disagreement per se does not mean that different scientific approaches or conclusions cannot be appealed to during the process of public justification. As long as scientists on either side of a dispute appeal to shared broad epistemic (scientific) standards, as long as none of them makes any gross epistemic error during their scientific inquiry, and as long as disagreement about factual standards (e.g. the relationship between eating and health) is the result of genuine scientific dispute, different approaches may provide grounds for publicly justified healthy eating efforts. For example, a healthy eating effort that aims specifically to reduce sodium intake or sugary drink

---

[4] For example, research concerning the beneficial health effects of cereal fibre found in whole and refined grains has revealed that 'the benefit was not found with cereal fiber from the endosperm [which can also be found in refined grains] but was found with the phytochemical-rich cereal fiber found in the whole grain, *when eaten as part of whole foods*' (Jacobs and Steffen 2003, p. 511S, emphasis added). Likewise, 'an apple, particularly with skin, contributes much more antioxidant capacity, from a wide variety of phytochemicals, than is available from its most studied constituent, vitamin C' (p. 512S). For an analysis of these debates, see Bonotti (2015).

consumption could be grounded in the view that sodium (or added sugar) is regularly consumed at levels that pose health risks; this would be reasonable. A different healthy eating effort could aim to promote consumption of 'whole foods' and could be grounded in the view that eating whole foods may have nutritional benefits that cannot be achieved simply by consuming the correct combination of nutrients; this would also be reasonable.

6.3.1.4. Industry money and self-interested science

The nutritionism debate points towards an interesting additional dimension of the process of public justification. Scrinis, we have seen, cites the role of the AND in this debate, and more specifically its critique of food-level nutritionism. However, some in the public health community do not find the AND credible, since it has received funding from such corporate groups as Kellogg's and Mars (Strom 2013).[5] This raises an important issue, which is the role of industry-funded research and the claims of industry in public justification. When researchers receive funding from industry actors to perform research, should we then discount their research findings for the purpose of public justification? Not necessarily. The source of research funding per se does not undermine the quality of scientific research. However, given the uncertainty surrounding nutrition research, there may be greater scope for actors with self-interested agendas to try to affect the direction and outcome of such research, or to draw on the findings of research in ways that may downplay the limits of the available empirical evidence and disagreements about it.

When industry actors appeal strategically to factual claims about which there is uncertainty and disagreement in order to advance their own sectarian interests, this is not acceptable for public justification. Indeed this kind of sectarianism is antithetical to public-mindedness and public reason (Gaus 2012) since it involves the promotion of the interests, values, and goals of specific individuals and groups within society, rather than the advancement

---

[5] Interestingly, as Scrinis points out, the food industry itself may sometimes actually embrace a nutritionist approach. More specifically, nutritionism has been used by the food industry over the past three decades as a framework to guide both the marketing of foods and diets on the one hand, and the production, processing, and re-engineering of foods on the other. A primary task of food scientists and technologists is to construct a nutritional façade around a food product, which becomes the focus of packaging and marketing strategies. Nutritionally marketed foods are explicitly promoted with nutrient-content claims on their labels or in advertisements, such as "low fat," "high protein," and "high in calcium." The marketing typically focuses on the absolute or relative quantities of one or two nutrients in the food, and in so doing, it tends to—often deliberately—distract attention from both the overall nutrient profile of a food and from the quality and characteristics of the food and its ingredients (Scrinis 2008, pp. 44–45).

of the common good. The sectarian use of true factual claims constitutes an infringement of the constraints of public reason even when those same factual claims would under different conditions be acceptable for public justification, e.g. when advanced in good faith as 'minority science' by someone who is acting with society's general interest in mind. That is, corporate actors who aim to advance their self-interest while also appealing to controversial factual beliefs are unreasonable, and they are acting differently from those public health policymakers who draw on controversial evidence in order to advance the general interest, aware that that evidence is imperfect but that sometimes this is the best we can hope for if we want to promote the common good.

6.3.1.5. Weak evidence for healthy eating efforts

A further issue concerns the *effects* of healthy eating efforts. We have so far mainly focused on the factual evidence concerning the relationship between body state and health, and between food consumption and health. But factual evidence also concerns the effectiveness of healthy eating efforts in tackling public health problems allegedly resulting from certain dietary patterns. One major concern with healthy eating efforts is that the evidence for efforts can be weak or mixed.

There are distinct ways in which the evidence base for healthy eating efforts can be weak. First, there may not be much evidence for a proposed policy; it simply has not been studied. Second, studies on healthy eating efforts may produce only weak evidence because of the nature of the research; e.g. nutrition studies may provide only weak evidence because research subjects do not follow a prescribed diet, or the research asks participants to recall and report what they ate but participants have low reliability. Third, the evidence base for a policy—even when there are a number of studies about it—might be mixed, with some evidence suggesting that the policy is effective and others suggesting that it is not (Fox and Horowitz 2013; Richardson et al. 2017; Williams 2015).

How can we address these problems within a public reason framework? When are these evidential issues a problem in connection with our accessibility standard? If the broad scientific methods that underlie the existing evidence are not shared (i.e. they are not those accepted by the scientific community), or if the specific conclusions reached (e.g. a claim about the effectiveness of a policy) are not justified in light of the existing evidence and shared scientific norms for its interpretation, then it seems unreasonable to proceed with a policy. But what if neither of these problems is at issue, and the evidence is simply mixed, e.g. because there is disagreement between different studies? Or there simply is not much evidence to evaluate, because the policy at issue has not been studied?

In these circumstances, policymakers may still have good reasons for enacting a policy despite a weak evidence base. This is because the strength of evidence necessary to justify a policy cannot be considered in isolation but should be examined instead in connection with the policy's potential benefits and burdens, and the evidence thereof. When the evidence for a policy is flawed, a policy should not be based on it. But when the available scientific evidence for a policy is simply weak (for the aforementioned reasons), a policymaker may recognize this but still have good reasons to go ahead with the policy based on that evidence; e.g. perhaps the public health problem at hand involves significant harm, and is urgent, and doing additional research would take too much time. We believe that this course of action is not unreasonable. While public justification must rely on science, science itself cannot determine public justification. Weak scientific evidence, as long as it is based on broadly shared scientific methods and does not result from gross epistemic error, can still provide valid grounds for public justification all things considered (i.e. once a policymaker has considered the importance and urgency of a situation).

In other words, whether or not a policy should be implemented despite weak evidence for its effectiveness *is* one of the questions that the process of public justification must address, rather than a question that should be answered before the process of public justification begins. That is, during the process of public justification regarding a proposed policy, one question that should be considered is whether the evidence base for the policy is sufficient. The consequences of delaying implementation of the policy are relevant to this question, as we have pointed out. Also relevant are the consequences of implementing the policy, and in particular its potential negative effects in light of important political values (e.g. citizens' equal basic liberties and rights). Nancy Kass (2001, pp. 1778–79) captures this latter point in her influential paper on the ethical analysis of public health programmes:

> While all programs must be based on sound data rather than informed speculation, the quality and volume of existing data will vary. The question for policy and ethics analysis, then, is what quantity of data is enough to justify a program's implementation? As a rule of thumb, the greater the

burdens posed by a program—for example, in terms of cost, constraints on liberty, or targeting particular, already vulnerable segments of the population—the stronger the evidence must be to demonstrate that the program will achieve its goals.

An interesting question is whether there are shared evaluative standards in the relevant expert communities (e.g. of scientists and/or policymakers) for establishing when the evidence for a policy is sufficient, and whether these standards about when evidence is sufficient are calibrated to moral benefits and burdens. Our hypothesis is that there are not such shared evaluative standards. In any case, we do not think that these are the kinds of standards that scientific experts should be allowed to determine. They belong to the domain of public justification, and, as we have already stressed, science can contribute to but should not determine the process of public justification, which involves many other considerations beyond scientific evidence.

6.3.1.6. Incomplete evidence about the (social, economic, and psycho-emotional) effects of healthy eating efforts

So far we have focused on issues concerning the natural science fact base for healthy eating efforts, e.g. disagreements about nutrition science, and the sometimes weak evidence base for the effectiveness of specific healthy eating efforts. But even if a policy is based on sound empirical evidence concerning its likely health effects, policymakers and the public may not have considered other important facts—i.e. facts about the broader social, psychological, and economic effects of the policy. We (policymakers and the public) may lack knowledge about the range of important social, psychological, and economic effects of healthy eating efforts. Arguably, the public health research community does not have a research programme in place to gather this kind of evidence about healthy eating efforts (Barnhill et al. 2018; Devine and Barnhill 2018).

One potential explanation for this is that those public health researchers and practitioners who are designing, implementing, and evaluating healthy eating efforts do not recognize that these efforts might have a range of social, psychological, and economic effects; this speaks to the need to have interdisciplinary teams, including social scientists, involved in the design and evaluation of healthy eating efforts. Another potential explanation for not gathering data on the social, psychological, and economic effects of healthy eating efforts is that these non-health effects of healthy eating efforts perhaps are not seen as relevant because the potential health benefits of those efforts are assigned overriding importance (what Mayes and Thompson [2014, p. 164] call 'characterizing eating occasions primarily in terms of nutritional or biomedical health'). On this explanation, healthy eating efforts reflect a kind of 'healthism'—treating health as 'a "super value" that trumps other social concerns' (Guthman 2011, Chap. 3; Mayes and Thompson 2014).

Another explanation, consistent with the others, is that some negative effects of healthy eating efforts are not salient because of various kinds of inequality; some people's experiences are overlooked or devalued. For example, scholars argue that women as a group expend significant effort on feeding work—planning and preparing meals, negotiating family members' food preferences, procuring food, cleaning up—but this effort is often overlooked or unacknowledged, or when it is acknowledged, it is devalued (Carrington 1999). Scholars have also argued that the work of mothers to promote their children's health (e.g. by feeding them healthy food) is often overlooked, and the costs to mothers of this work are not acknowledged, perhaps because we have the normative expectation of mothers that they will sacrifice their own interests in order to provide even a modest amount of benefit to their children (an 'ethic of total motherhood'), and thus it is not notable when mothers make these sacrifices (Wolf 2010). In an analogous way, the negative effects of healthy eating efforts on other systematically disadvantaged groups (low-income people, racial and ethnic minority groups, etc.) may be overlooked or devalued.

Healthy eating efforts are unreasonable—they are not publicly justified—if they fail to take into account relevant facts concerning their social, psychological, and economic effects on people. The failure to take these facts into account may result in worse (e.g. less effective) efforts, since interventions with unrecognized (and therefore unmitigated) negative effects may not get uptake with the target population or may not be sustainable (Devine and Barnhill 2018). Furthermore, neglecting relevant social, psychological, and economic facts raises moral concerns. First, this neglect may be driven by various forms of injustice, and especially of *epistemic* injustice (Fricker 2007). More specifically, it could involve a form of hermeneutical injustice, i.e. a 'structural prejudice in the economy of collective hermeneutical resources' (p. 1). This kind of injustice occurs when a society lacks the collective interpretative resources necessary for a group to understand (and express) key aspects of their social experience, or when a group's reports on their own experience are not treated as authoritative. The way in which policymakers often neglect to consider the effects of healthy eating efforts may fit this model: those negatively affected by healthy eating efforts may lack the epistemic resources to fully understand and express their situation or the political power to make their voices heard, or those designing such efforts may fail to take them seriously.

Furthermore, when public policy neglects the potential economic, social, and psychological effects of healthy eating efforts, those efforts will be illegitimate and publicly unjustified. For example, if efforts neglect or assign insufficient importance to people's personal values associated with eating and/or health, or make it particularly difficult for them to pursue their life plans and conceptions of the good, then these efforts overly burden them. It would therefore be illegitimate to impose such efforts upon them. This point is captured by Rawls' (1999, p. 153) idea of the 'strains of commitment', which is succinctly summarized by Quong (2006, pp. 59–60) in the following way:

> Although laws should be impartial in terms of their justification and not necessarily in their consequences, it's important to be clear about what justificatory impartiality requires. Non-discriminatory intent is a necessary but not sufficient condition of justificatory impartiality. There are many laws that might meet the condition of being non-discriminatory in their intent, yet would clearly be unjustifiable on account of the unreasonable burdens they impose on certain persons. Justificatory neutrality requires not just that we avoid discriminatory intent, but also that we imagine what impact a given policy will have on all affected parties. We fail to reason impartially if we don't consider how the burdens and benefits of a policy will be distributed. In addition to the condition of non-discriminatory intent, impartial justification requires something along the lines of Rawls's 'strains of commitment' condition. I fail to reason impartially if I support a policy whose burdens and benefits are distributed in such a way that I wouldn't agree to place myself in the position of those who are worst-off under the policy.

In some cases, therefore, healthy eating efforts are unjustified and illegitimate because their foreseeable effects may impose disproportionate burdens on certain citizens. This does not mean, of course, that *any* negative effects healthy eating efforts may have on some people entail that those efforts are not publicly justified. After all, our accessibility view of public reason aims precisely to offer a public justification for healthy eating efforts despite the fact that the latter may be in tension with some people's beliefs, values, and preferences. However, when being 'worst-off under the [healthy eating] policy' means not being able to pursue one's life plan (or being able to do so only at an excessive or unreasonable cost), and/or when those suffering from the disproportionate burdens resulting from a healthy eating effort are mainly members of an already disadvantaged group (which may also suffer from the disproportionate burdens resulting from other policies, perhaps due to structural injustice), then we are in the presence of strains of commitment that undermine the public justification for the policy. This discussion suggests that while it is necessary for healthy eating efforts to be justified by appealing to facts about their health effects, this is not sufficient. It is also necessary that public justification for these efforts does not neglect other relevant facts, e.g. facts about those efforts' *other* (i.e. non-health) effects.

6.3.2. Examples of descriptive metaphysical evaluative standards in healthy eating policy debate

In the previous section we focused on what we call factual evaluative standards and prescriptive epistemic evaluative standards. We showed that sometimes healthy eating efforts may be justified by appealing to factual evidence that is weak or controversial, i.e. not fully shared amongst members of the scientific community and/or the general public. We pointed out that this is almost inevitable, given the complexity of the relationships between food and health. However, we stressed that appealing to controversial facts is reasonable if these are established by using epistemic evaluative standards that are broadly shared by scientists (and, in principle, by members of the public) in liberal societies, and if no gross epistemic error is made in the process. We also highlighted the importance that other factors play in the use of factual evidence during the process of public justification. More specifically, even when empirical evidence is controversial or weak, it may be acceptable for policymakers to appeal to it if this is the best that can be achieved given practical constraints, and if the goal is to promote shared political values. Furthermore, we pointed out that the weighing and selection of factual evidence may be influenced by the interests of different actors, e.g. the food industry, and that this may sometimes result in unreasonable justifications for healthy eating efforts.

In the present section we focus on the third category of evaluative standards illustrated earlier, i.e. descriptive metaphysical beliefs. These, we have seen, include controversial religious beliefs or beliefs related to supernatural or folk worldviews, though they also include broadly shared beliefs, e.g. beliefs concerning the identity of persons and the persistence of objects over time. The key feature of these kinds of evaluative standards is that, unlike factual evaluative standards, they cannot be established via scientific inquiry.

What interest us in this section are controversial metaphysical beliefs which may generate inaccessible reasons and therefore potentially undermine the public justification of healthy eating efforts. Admittedly, it may be rare to find healthy eating efforts grounded in these kinds of inaccessible reasons. However, such reasons are more relevant when it comes to some individuals' and groups' *opposition* to healthy eating efforts. We explained in the previous chapter that the intelligibility conception of public reason allows individuals to advance reasons, based on their religious or otherwise controversial views, that defeat healthy eating efforts. When it comes to accessibility, however, we saw that as long as policies are based on accessible reasons, they can be permissibly implemented even if many citizens object to them.

The problem, though, is that accessibility still requires that the evaluative standards a public reason relies on are evaluative standards that are widely shared in that society. Now, in the high-income liberal democracies that are the focus of this book, we can assume that belief in the evaluative standards of science is widespread, whereas supernatural and religious evaluative standards are highly controversial (Badano and Bonotti 2020). This determines the extent to which healthy eating efforts can be justified by appealing to reasons grounded in either type of evaluative standards. Different kinds of evaluative standards, however, may be predominant in different societies. For example, a recent study showed that in Ethiopia adherence to pregnancy-related food taboos is widespread and results in high rates of maternal anemia (Mohammed et al. 2019). On our taxonomy, taboos are metaphysical (rather than descriptive factual) evaluative standards, since they cannot be established via scientific inquiry. In the Ethiopian context, the fact that adherence to pregnancy-related food taboos is widespread means that public health policymakers may struggle to appeal to certain factual scientific claims to justify healthy eating efforts, if such claims are in tension with the metaphysical beliefs held by many citizens, which may prevent the latter from believing in those scientific conclusions. This kind of conflict may also be present in other societies, including the high-income liberal democracies that are our focus. Indeed, as Badano and Bonotti (2020, p. 62) point out:

> An argument can be controversial, even if it is undisputed among scientifically-minded persons, if a person cannot accept it as their own because of the sheer tension with strongly-held beliefs they hold as part of their comprehensive doctrine. This understanding of the potentially controversial character of scientific arguments seems to capture, at least in part, what underlies the public rejection of scientific opinions in some important controversies. For example, some people reject arguments from evolutionary biology because these arguments cannot possibly fit with deeply-held beliefs in their comprehensive doctrines (which might be very strongly invested in the divine creation of all living beings, in intelligent design, etc.).

However, at least in most high-income liberal democracies, this tension may not provide a decisive argument against the public justifiability of state policies (including healthy eating efforts), since science retains its status as a source of truth for most people, even if many people also consider religion a source of truth (see Badano and Bonotti 2020). But can this widespread belief in science as a source of truth be ascribed to all societies? If not, can policymakers rely on the conclusions of science in those societies where such conclusions are in conflict with many citizens' metaphysical beliefs? Here, a number of different answers might be possible.

First, one might argue that if policymakers aim to promote the common good in the form of public health (a shared moral evaluative standard in all societies, we can assume), it may be permissible for them to appeal to scientific facts that conflict with many citizens' beliefs. But it is not clear why this might be the case. If the public political culture of a society does not involve a widespread belief in the value of science, it is not clear how accessible public reasons may rely on such beliefs.[6] Alternatively, one might contend that idealized versions of citizens of all societies might recognize the value of science, but arguably this involves an excessive level of idealization. Another answer is that unlike political values, which are relative to specific societies and their

---

[6] The same conclusion would apply to societies where widespread belief in science is currently prevalent, if these were to gradually move away from a widespread belief in the value of science.

political cultures, the methods and conclusions of science are universal. But can we make this kind of argument within the framework of public reason liberalism that we have sketched, which yokes public justification in a particular society to the moral and epistemic values central to that society's public political culture?

A better answer might be that we should not view public reasoning as a static process. Public reason can change (Flanders 2012), i.e. the evaluative standards that are shared in a society can evolve, thus also changing the shared vocabulary of public justification in that society. That change, as Flanders observes, may happen via what Rawls calls the 'background culture' of society, i.e. the 'culture of churches and associations of all kinds, and institutions of learning at all levels, *especially universities and professional schools, scientific and other societies*' (Rawls 2005a, p. 443, note 13, emphasis added). It may be the case that, with time, scientific institutions in societies where belief in science is not widespread will contribute to changing that trend, thus rendering appeals to science in support of policymaking more widely accepted.

Finally, it should also be noted that in some cases religious, supernatural, and folk metaphysical beliefs about food, such as those that underlie some food taboos, in fact conceal sound scientific and medical beliefs about those foods (Meyer-Rochow 2009). In such cases there may not be a tension between metaphysical and scientific beliefs. As long as those metaphysical beliefs about food are grounded in scientific evidence, and as long as their scientific roots are acknowledged, they may therefore be included in the process of public justification (they are indirectly accessible, so to speak).

6.3.2.1. Unreasonable judgements about foods' healthfulness

The mutability of public reason examined in the previous section is potentially a double-edged sword. While a widespread belief in science may emerge in societies where it is currently not present, that widespread belief may also gradually weaken in a society. That could be a problem for the role of science in public justification. This shows the important role that universities and other scientific and educational institutions can play in ensuring that scientific methods and conclusions remain widely endorsed amongst citizens, even amongst those who also embrace religious or other controversial metaphysical beliefs.

But even without imagining this radical change, and even if we continue to assume that most societies, including the high-income liberal democracies that are the focus of our book, display a widespread belief in science, we can still witness instances of controversial beliefs being used to justify various types of healthy eating efforts in those societies. For example, metaphysical beliefs about the 'natural' (e.g. the view that organic foods are natural and therefore healthier) are widespread in many societies. Empirical research has found that people prefer entities perceived to be or described as 'natural', e.g. natural foods. People perceive natural entities to have specific advantages, such as being healthier, better for the environment, more pleasant, and purer and safer (Li and Chapman 2012; Rozin et al. 2004). Likewise, DiBonaventura and Chapman (2008, p. 2) identify what they call 'naturalness bias', i.e. 'the tendency to prefer natural products or substances even when they are identical to or worse than synthetic alternatives'. DiBonaventura and Chapman identify naturalness bias in opposition to genetically modified foods, but claims about the natural also appear in discussions of a wide range of other issues in health, science, and technology, including childhood vaccination, alternative medicine, assisted reproduction, cloning, stem cell research, agriculture and food, and 'natural' products (Nuffield Council on Bioethics 2015).

When a connection is drawn between naturalness and healthfulness, this connection may sometimes be justified (e.g. if 'natural' is just being used to mean 'nutritionally suitable'). However, in other cases the connection between naturalness and healthfulness is not justified, or at least it is controversial (Siipi 2013). For example, there is evidence that natural entities are perceived by some people to be *inherently* better, morally and aesthetically: when study participants are told that a natural entity has the same properties (taste, healthfulness, etc.) as an unnatural version, or is chemically identical to an unnatural version, some retain a preference for the natural version (Rozin et al. 2004). To the extent that the preference for natural foods is grounded in moral, aesthetic, or other ideational reasons, it therefore belongs to the category of metaphysical evaluative standards, since naturalness thus intended cannot be established via scientific inquiry. If appeals to naturalness as a metaphysical evaluative standard were made in the defence of healthy eating efforts, and assuming that such a standard is not widely shared, those efforts would be unreasonable. For example, imagine a hypothetical policy that subsidized the purchase of fresh produce from local farmers markets but did not subsidize the purchase of canned and frozen produce from local grocery stores. Suppose that someone advocates for this policy by arguing that the fresh fruits and vegetables grown by local farmers are more 'natural' and therefore better than the frozen and canned produce available in local grocery stores; this would not be a reasonable defence of the policy and should be excluded from public justification. However, other defences of the policy could be given that are reasonable, e.g. arguing that the policy supports local farmers engaged in sustainable agriculture and that this will be good for the local economy and environment.

Li and Chapman (2012) call Rozin et al.'s (2004) findings into question, and suggest that beliefs in the *instrumental* (as opposed to *inherent*) benefits of natural entities may not have been detected by some previous work. They find that study participants are reluctant to believe that natural and unnatural entities really pose the same risk, or really are identical, even when the study specifies that they are. Thus, what looks like a preference for the natural because it is inherently better (i.e. a metaphysical or moral belief) may actually be a preference rooted in the unshakeable belief that natural options have specific functional advantages (i.e. an incorrect belief about a scientific fact). In such cases, appeals to the naturalness of certain foods in the public justification of healthy eating efforts will still be unreasonable. However, these appeals will be unreasonable not because they are based on metaphysical evaluative standards but because they are grounded in pseudo-science or bad science, something that violates prescriptive epistemic and/or descriptive factual evaluative standards.

6.3.3. Examples of prescriptive moral evaluative standards in healthy eating policy debate

In this final section we discuss prescriptive moral evaluative standards. We explained earlier in this chapter that these include shared political values such as basic rights and liberties as well as equality of opportunity, the absence of structural injustice, and the common good. What, then, are the main ways in which healthy eating efforts can promote shared political values?

As we have stressed previously in this book, healthy eating efforts can promote citizens' health, and this can help them to fully enjoy their basic rights and liberties (Rawls 2005a, p. 228)[7] as well as access to a greater range of opportunities (Daniels 2008). Healthy eating efforts can also help to promote health equity—i.e. to reduce health inequalities between social groups that

---

[7] See also Kaufman (2018, pp. 223–24).

are unjust, such as higher rates of diet-related illness in some communities of colour. They can also help to promote individuals' well-being and their exercise of the second moral power, i.e. 'the capacity to form, to revise and rationally to pursue a conception of one's rational advantage or good' (Rawls 2005a, p. 19). Furthermore, they can help advance the common good, e.g. because a healthier society is economically more prosperous.

Sometimes, we have seen, there may be disagreement regarding the meaning and scope of these shared political values. For example, there could be disagreement about what equality of opportunity requires when it comes to healthy eating; e.g. does it require just that all people can afford healthy food (though they might have to make other sacrifices), or does it require that all people can *easily* afford healthy food, or does it require that healthy food is cheap enough that most people actually prefer to buy and consume a healthy diet over a less healthy one? There could also be disagreement about what racial equity requires; e.g. does it require equal health outcomes across all racial/ethnic groups, equal access to healthy food, equal control over shaping healthy eating policy, or something else? This disagreement about the precise interpretations and applications of shared political values that are appealed to in order to justify healthy eating efforts will not necessarily result in healthy eating efforts being unreasonable. As Rawls (2005b, p. 450) points out, political liberalism allows 'a family of political conceptions of justice', each involving different specifications of key political values.

Yet, our intuition is that the scope for reasonable interpretations of shared political values cannot be unlimited. For example, freedom of speech is a widely shared political value in liberal democratic societies, and most people agree that freedom of speech covers political speech, since the latter is considered a fundamental prerogative of citizens in a democratic system. Yet, the belief that commercial speech by business enterprises falls within the scope of freedom of speech is (arguably) a much more controversial interpretation of that freedom. Thus, if a proposal for a healthy eating effort involving modest restrictions on food marketing is objected to or reversed on the grounds that it violates freedom of speech, this may be unreasonable. Not all interpretations of shared political values are reasonable. Some, more than others, may explicitly or implicitly be grounded in the interests of specific individuals or groups (e.g. corporations) within society, rather than in arguments that appeal to the common good, thus reintroducing through the back door the kind of sectarianism that political liberalism and its ideal of public justification aimed to eschew.

A more common scenario, perhaps, is one in which healthy eating efforts are grounded in reasons that overly prioritize certain shared political values or neglect others. Healthy eating efforts that do so are not publicly justified under the accessibility conception since they are grounded in an unreasonable balance of political values (Quong 2011, p. 207). An example of neglecting shared political values would be if policymakers designed healthy eating efforts to promote the common good (e.g. to maximize public health benefit and economic benefit) without paying attention to whether the efforts disproportionately burden certain groups, thus generating the aforementioned strains of commitment. For example, some healthy eating efforts may impose excessive burdens specifically on women (e.g. campaigns encouraging healthy eating at home) given their disproportionate share of feeding work. Another example of neglecting shared political values is if policymakers fail to consider racial inequity when designing healthy eating efforts, and fail to consider the higher rates of diet-related illness in some communities of colour, or fail to consider the ways in which higher rates of diet-related illness reflect background structural racism and thus require remedy. In these examples, healthy eating efforts are not publicly justified since they neglect the foreseeable strains of commitment they may impose upon women and communities of colour. And this amounts to neglecting or assigning insufficient importance to the shared political values of gender and racial equality, since failing to consider how the burdens and benefits of a policy will be distributed risks compounding existing structural injustices along these dimensions.

Another example of neglecting political values is if policymakers assume that consumption of an unhealthy food has no value for individuals, without considering how it might feature in people's life plans or provide value for them—in effect, ignoring the value of individuals exercising their second moral power, i.e. forming, revising, and pursuing their own conception of the good.

Likewise, designers and supporters of healthy eating efforts neglect certain shared political values if they ignore or assign insufficient importance to individual freedom and consumer choice when designing and justifying those efforts—e.g. if supporters of a product ban do not take seriously the fact that the ban limits consumers' liberty and limits the liberty of companies to market products, or if they denigrate this liberty as obviously unimportant. Vice versa, another way of neglecting certain political values is if policymakers assume that individual consumer freedom has overriding importance, and it should always be prioritized over the common good and over various justice goals, and thus policymakers should reject any healthy eating efforts that limit consumer choice (Beauchamp 1976, 1980).[8] Always prioritizing economic freedoms can be particularly problematic; while such freedoms are certainly important in a liberal democracy, they are arguably less important than other freedoms (e.g. freedom of speech or freedom of religion) from the perspective of political liberalism (Freeman 2007, pp. 56ff). Therefore, economic freedoms may often permissibly be sacrificed for the realization of political values that healthy eating efforts can help realize, such as equality of opportunity, the common good, or the protection and advancement of more fundamental liberties and rights.

The problem of guaranteeing a reasonable balance of political values also involves the kind of evidential issues highlighted in the previous section. More specifically, often the balance that needs to be achieved in order for a healthy eating effort to be reasonable is not only between different political values. Instead, it also concerns balancing different political values in relation to different levels of empirical evidence. That is, when certain healthy eating efforts are implemented, this will *certainly* result in a reduction of, say, liberty (e.g. food bans) or equity and fairness (e.g. sugary drink taxes or fast food taxes that are more of a financial burden on lower-income people). At the same time, it may be *uncertain* whether the efforts will work. Considering a healthy eating effort publicly justified under these conditions therefore seems to imply a moral judgement of the following kind: an unknown chance to promote health (and its contribution to shared political values) for all citizens justifies a 100% chance of reducing liberty or equity and fairness for some citizens. This requires some guidelines for assessing when healthy eating efforts are reasonable, taking into account all four kinds of evaluative standards examined in this chapter. It is to the development of such a framework that we turn in Chapter 7.

---

[8] While Rawls assigns priority to basic liberties such as freedom of thought, conscience, speech, and association, over the common good and socio-economic justice, individual consumer freedom is not a basic liberty and therefore does not deserve this kind of protection—i.e. it can be traded off against other (non-liberty) values.

7

Designing Publicly Justified Healthy Eating Efforts

7.1. Introduction

In this book we have defended a liberal approach to healthy eating policy that is grounded in the ideals of public justification and public reason. Healthy eating efforts, we have claimed, should be normatively assessed not based on whether they reflect one kind of value or moral orientation (e.g. whether they are paternalistic or anti-paternalistic) but based on whether they can be publicly justified by appealing to accessible public reasons. This approach, we have contended, can help policymakers implement healthy eating efforts that are politically legitimate in spite of the pluralism of conceptions of the good (including conceptions of health and eating) that characterizes contemporary diverse liberal societies.

Based on our analysis, in this final chapter we provide guidance to help public health policymakers navigate the complex empirical and moral issues surrounding healthy eating policy illustrated in the previous chapters. First, we sketch a 'public reason framework for healthy eating efforts' that public health officials, legislators, and others can use to assess proposed or existing healthy eating efforts. This framework consists of questions that public health officials and legislators should ask themselves when designing new healthy eating efforts or evaluating existing ones with an eye toward reforming or repealing them if necessary. These questions are grounded in the ideal of public reason, as presented in this book. Second, we make recommendations about institutionalizing the use of this framework (and, by extension, institutionalizing the public justification of healthy eating efforts) by incorporating into policymaking a process of consultation and deliberation that includes public health officials, ordinary citizens, advocacy groups, and representatives of affected groups.

Healthy Eating Policy and Political Philosophy. Anne Barnhill and Matteo Bonotti, Oxford University Press. © Oxford University Press 2022. DOI: 10.1093/oso/9780190937881.003.0008

7.2. Ethics frameworks for public health

The framework we present in this chapter is an example of an *ethics tool*. Ethics tools are practical tools that aim to improve decision-making by systematically incorporating ethical considerations and structuring ethical reflection. Ethics tools come in different forms (flowcharts, checklists, lists of questions, matrices, and methods for guiding group discussion and deliberation), are designed for use by different actors (clinicians, public health professionals, policymakers, stakeholder groups, etc.), are focused on different topic areas (e.g. public health, clinical medicine, biomedical research, and agrifood issues), and are used in multiple ways (to help decision-makers think through the ethics of specific policies, practices, or decisions; to canvass the opinions of stakeholders to inform decisions; and to communicate the ethical basis of decisions) (Beekman et al. 2006; Beekman and Brom 2007; Bremer et al. 2016; Deblonde et al. 2007; Faden et al. 2013; Kass 2001; Lee 2012; Mepham 2000; ten Have et al. 2013).

Our ethics framework draws on existing ethics frameworks for public health, and in particular Childress et al. (2002), Kass (2001), and ten Have et al. (2013).[1] These frameworks offer public health practitioners (and other framework users) guidance on navigating the ethical challenges that they face in designing public health programmes and policies that are ethically justifiable.

Kass (2001) offers an elegant ethics framework for public health programmes which helps users assess the ethics of a proposed public health programme or policy by asking and answering a series of questions about it (Figure 7.1). In essence, Kass's framework guides the user through a structured process of ethical reasoning about the policy under consideration. Our framework, as we will see, has the same basic form.

Ten Have et al. (2013) offer an ethics framework focused specifically on obesity prevention programmes. Similar to Kass's framework, theirs guides the user through a structured process of ethical reasoning, which includes the following steps: identifying the policy's ethical strengths and drawbacks along multiple dimensions (e.g. informed choice, equality, psychosocial wellbeing, social and cultural values); considering ways to minimize drawbacks and maximize strengths, and whether there is an alternative with fewer ethical drawbacks; considering whether the policy's ethical drawbacks can be

---

[1] See Lee (2012) for a helpful overview of multiple ethics frameworks for public health.

To ethically assess a public health programme, ask the following questions about it:

(1) What are the public health goals of the proposed programme?

(2) How effective is the programme in achieving its stated goals?

(3) What are the known or potential burdens of the programme?

(4) Can burdens be minimized? Are there alternative approaches?

(5) Is the programme implemented fairly?

(6) How can the benefits and burdens of the programme be fairly balanced?

Figure 7.1 Kass's (2001) ethics framework for public health.

justified; and defining 'whether and under what conditions the programme is acceptable from an ethical point of view' (p. 304). A welcome feature of ten Have et al.'s framework, and one that is well-aligned with our perspective on healthy eating policy, is that the framework draws the user's attention to various distinct kinds of ethical drawbacks that obesity prevention programmes may have, e.g. potential negative effects on psychosocial well-being, social and cultural values, liberty, and equality. Helpfully, the framework also suggests that groups of people should use it to assess policies and offers guidance about the numbers and kinds of participants who should be included in this group process.

All three ethics frameworks we draw on recognize that there will be diverse perspectives on public health efforts and that this necessitates seeking public input into policy design and assessment, having fair decision-making processes, and providing normative justifications for these efforts. For example, Kass (2001, p. 1781) writes:

And yet while most reasonable people will agree, in the abstract, that burdens and benefits must be balanced, and that the most burdensome programs should be implemented only in the context of extensive and important benefits, disagreements are all but guaranteed over the details. Depending on one's perspective, there will be differing views over how burdensome various programs are, such as having one's name reported to the state or being required to immunize children before they start school . . . Solutions to these inevitable disagreements must be reached through a system of fair procedures. Procedural justice requires a society to engage in a democratic process to determine which public health functions it wants its government to maintain, recognizing that some infringements of liberty and other burdens are unavoidable. There should be open discussion of what a society gains from good public health and why such benefits often cannot be obtained through less communal or more liberty-preserving methods. The discussion, of course, should also address why other interests also have moral claim. Such a process, even when procedurally fair by most standards, must not result in decisions based solely on the will of the majority. Indeed, deliberations, particularly around significantly burdensome proposals, must be scrutinized to ensure that the views of the minority are given due consideration.

Childress et al. (2002) incorporate public justification and public reason into their framework, albeit in a somewhat vague way. They argue that when public health efforts infringe on important moral considerations (e.g. liberty or privacy), public health officials must offer public justification for those efforts:

> When public health agents believe that one of their actions, practices, or policies infringes one or more general moral considerations, they also have a responsibility, in our judgment, to explain and justify that infringement, whenever possible, to the relevant parties, including those affected by the infringement. In the context of what we called 'political public', public health agents should offer public justification for policies in terms that fit the overall social contract in a liberal, pluralistic democracy. This transparency stems in part from the requirement to treat citizens as equals and with respect by offering moral reasons, which in principle they could find acceptable, for policies that infringe general moral considerations. (p. 173)

We are in agreement with Childress et al. that public justification is required for public health efforts that infringe moral considerations (and for public health efforts in general, we would add). Our framework is meant to provide guidance on how to incorporate public reason and public justification into public health policy in a detailed way. Successfully achieving public justification requires careful attention to the kinds of reasons offered for public health efforts and requires filtering out non-public reasons. We should not expect that public health officials or other actors assessing policies will know a priori how to do this; our framework provides them with guidance in doing so.

7.3. Public reason and a 'principlist' approach to practical ethics

Ethics frameworks such as those developed by Childress et al. (2002), Kass (2001), and ten Have et al. (2013) can be seen as broadly employing 'principlism', a dominant methodology in bioethics. As developed by Beauchamp and Childress (2019) in their hugely influential *The Principles of Biomedical Ethics*, first published in 1979, the methodology of principlism starts with multiple broad ethical principles and values that are relevant to specific domains. For example, Beauchamp and Childress identify four broad ethical principles for the biomedical domain: autonomy, beneficence (promoting good or preventing harm), non-maleficence (not causing harm), and justice. In particular instances, when one is ethically assessing a particular policy or action, one must figure out how those broad ethical principles apply to the specific instance at hand (a process called 'specification'). As it turns out, there might be conflicts between the principles; e.g. 'autonomy' may call for making sure that your patient is fully informed about the risks of the surgery you are recommending, whereas 'beneficence' may call for glossing over those risks if disclosing them in detail would deter the patient from consenting to a surgery that offers her far more benefit than harm. When ethical principles are in tension or conflict, these ethical principles must be *balanced.*

The methodology of principlism and our approach to public reason are broadly aligned. Both involve recognizing, first, that a range of values is at stake with any given policy decision; second, that these values may conflict; and third, that these values may need to be balanced. The distinctiveness of our approach in this book is that we draw on political philosophy to provide a specific theoretical justification and grounding for a broadly principlist approach to the normative assessment of healthy eating policy. That is, we are grounding a principlist approach to the normative assessment of healthy eating policy in a specific account of public reason and public justification.

On this 'public reason' grounding of a principlist approach to assessing public policy, the principlist approach has certain distinctive features. Public justification must be given for public health policies and programmes, and there are certain kinds of values or reasons (non-public reasons) that should not be included in the public justification of policies and programmes. Therefore, the framework provides criteria for the 'filtering out' of reasons grounded in values that are controversial and non-political, e.g. those grounded in sectarian interests or controversial religious and ethical doctrines, as well as reasons grounded in an unreasonable balance of political values. Furthermore, our public reason approach includes an epistemic dimension: public justification for healthy eating efforts must be grounded both in a reasonable balance of shared political values and in sound empirical evidence, and the relationship between these two conditions is complex, as we explained in Chapter 6.

7.4. Our framework

Our framework has three main goals. First, the process that it outlines aims to guarantee the public justification of healthy eating efforts. This process, and the questions central to it, are based on our accessibility conception of public reason. The framework's questions guide the user through a process of identifying the aims and potential unintended side effects of a policy (and the evidence for them), considering how these aims and side effects promote or hinder political values, and considering whether the policy strikes a reasonable balance of political values. The framework is meant to help the user avoid the shortcomings illustrated in Chapter 6. Second, the framework aims to render public health policymakers more accountable to the ordinary citizens for whom healthy eating efforts are intended, by making policymakers more responsive to the latter's needs, interests, and value preferences. Third, the framework intends to contribute to the implementation of more effective healthy eating efforts. When efforts are publicly justified in ways that take into account people's needs, interests, and values, they are not only more legitimate but may also be more effective. Understanding in a detailed way how policies affect people will presumably allow policymakers to design more effective policies.

Having outlined the rationale for our framework, we will now illustrate its key elements (Figure 7.2). We present these in the form of questions that public health practitioners or others ought to ask themselves when designing or (re-)evaluating healthy eating efforts.

7.4.1 What are the public health-related aims of the policy?

The framework's first main question is the following: (1) *What are the public health–related aims of the policy?* Answering this question will require

1. What are the public health-related aims of the policy?

　　(a) How likely is it that the policy will achieve its stated public health-related aims?

　　(b) If the policy achieves its aims, will this advance shared political values and, if so, which ones?

(2) Does the policy have other (non-public-health-related) aims?

　　(a) How likely is it that the policy will achieve these other aims?

　　(b) Do these non-public-health-related aims advance shared political values and, if so, how?

　　(c) Do these non-public-health-related aims advance controversial non-political values and, if so, how?

(3) Is the policy likely to have any unintended positive or negative side effects?

　　(a) How likely is it that the policy will have these side effects?

　　(b) Do these effects advance shared political values and, if so, how?

　　(c) Do these side effects hinder shared political values and/or advance controversial non-political values and, if so, how?

(4) Does the policy strike a reasonable balance of political values?

　　(a) If not, can it be modified so that it does?

When addressing these questions, users should consider:

　　(i) how they (or other kinds of professionals, experts, or advocates) would answer them
　　(ii) how a typical member of the public/community (or communities) targeted or affected by the policy would answer them (and, if there are several relevant distinct groups, how a typical member of each of them would answer them)
　　(iii) how someone with a worldview or ideology different from theirs (and, more generally, from the view(s) that is/are dominant among policymakers) would answer them
　　(iv) if there is disagreement between these three answers to a question, how a fair-minded group of people who are listening to everyone's point of view, but also trying to reach agreement, would resolve this issue.

Figure 7.2 A public reason framework for healthy eating efforts

explaining what specific, proximate outcomes a healthy eating policy aims to achieve and, if these are not health outcomes, how these proximate outcomes will lead to or contribute to health outcomes. These proximate outcomes might include specific changes in attitudes (e.g. increased knowledge about the sugar content of purchased food), changes in purchasing behaviour (e.g. reduced purchases of sugary drinks) or changes in consumption (e.g. reduced consumption of added sugars, reduced sodium intake, increased consumption of fruits and vegetables). The health outcomes that these proximate outcomes are expected to lead to, or contribute to, might include reduced rates of diabetes, high blood pressure, or cardiovascular disease as well as weight maintenance, weight loss, or reductions in rates of overweight or obesity. In some cases, a policy will aim to achieve an outcome in a particular population, e.g. reducing sugary drink consumption amongst adolescents or reducing diabetes amongst Black residents of a city.

Policymakers will then need to ask two additional questions. First, (a) *How likely is it that the policy will achieve its stated public health–related aims?* In other words, what is the evidence for the effectiveness of the policy? For example, how likely is it that introducing a sugary drink tax will reduce the purchase of sugary drinks in the jurisdiction where the tax applies, that this reduction in purchases in that jurisdiction will translate into a reduction in total consumption of sugary drinks by any population, and that this reduction in total consumption of sugary drinks will ultimately have health benefits? Are these predictions based on sound scientific evidence (or, on the contrary, on flawed data and/or gross epistemic errors)? Addressing these questions will require (i) gathering any existing scientific evidence concerning the policy's likelihood of achieving its aims; (ii) considering the amount and quality of this evidence; (iii) excluding from consideration any evidence that is based on flawed data and/or gross epistemic errors; and (iv) ascertaining whether there is scientific consensus about the remaining evidence and its interpretation (and, if not, what the majority and minority positions are). When such evidence does not exist yet, policymakers might consider commissioning new research to investigate the potential effectiveness of the policy.

Second, (b) *If the policy achieves its aims, will this advance shared political values, and, if so, which ones?* For example, does the policy aim to improve health in order to improve people's enjoyment of their basic rights and liberties? Or to address health inequities rooted in systemic racism? Or to advance equality of opportunity? Or to reduce healthcare costs and advance the common good? If the evidence for either the policy's effectiveness or its contribution to political values (or both) is weak, policymakers should then consider whether the policy is justifiable despite weak evidence. If a policy addresses a public health problem involving significant harm, and one that urgently requires action, then the policy may be justifiable despite weak evidence. If it is not, then policymakers should consider whether it can be modified into a policy for which there is stronger evidence and/or which is more likely to advance shared political values; if that it is not possible, they should consider whether this provides grounds for rejecting the policy.

7.4.2 Does the policy have other aims?

The framework's second main question is the following: (2) *Does the policy have other (non-public-health-related) aims?* Answering this question will require explaining what non-public-health-related aims (if any) the relevant healthy eating policy aims to achieve. These might include, e.g., providing people with resources (e.g. more food assistance), raising revenue, creating jobs, supporting local farmers, or spurring economic revitalization. Policymakers will then need to ask three additional questions.

First, (a) *How likely is it that the policy will achieve these other aims?* In other words, what is the evidence for the effectiveness of the policy with regard to these aims? For example, suppose that the policy under consideration is a proposed sugary drink tax, and one of its non-health aims is to raise significant revenue. How likely is it that introducing this tax will raise significant revenue? And are these predictions based on sound scientific evidence (or, on the contrary, based on flawed data and/or gross epistemic errors)? Once again, addressing these questions will require (i) gathering any existing scientific evidence concerning the policy's likelihood of achieving its aims; (ii) considering the amount and quality of this evidence; and (iii) ascertaining whether there is scientific consensus about this evidence (and, if not, what the majority and minority positions are). When such evidence does not exist yet, policymakers might consider commissioning new research to investigate the potential effectiveness of the policy.

Second, (b) *Do these other aims advance shared political values, and, if so, how?* For example, will creating more jobs increase equality of opportunity? Will providing people with more resources help to address various forms of injustice?

Third, (c) *Do these other aims hinder shared political values and/or advance controversial non-political values and, if so, how?* For example, is the aim of economic revitalization intended to favour the sectarian interests of specific economic actors? Do certain politicians or parties aim to use the extra tax revenue to their own sectarian advantage?

If the evidence of the policy's likely effectiveness in achieving its non-health aims or contributing to shared political values (or both) is weak, policymakers might consider rejecting the policy or modifying it in such a way that it meets the two desiderata. When the justification for a policy turns out to be grounded in non-political sectarian aims and values, policymakers should either try to find public reasons for the same policy or, if these are not available, modify the policy in such a way that it can be justified by appealing to public reasons. If this is not possible, the policy should be rejected. For example, could a sugary drink tax be designed in such a way that the tax revenue will be allocated to activities that clearly advance shared political values rather than favouring specific sectarian interests? As a concrete example of this, when the city of Philadelphia, Pennsylvania, passed a sugary drink tax in 2017, it allocated revenue to providing public funding for early childhood education (which advances equality of opportunity) and for schools, parks, libraries, and recreation centres (which broadly advance equality of opportunity and the common good).

7.4.3 Is the policy likely to have unintended effects?

The framework's third main question is the following: (3) *Is the policy likely to have any unintended positive or negative side effects, and, if so, (a) How likely is it that the policy will have these side effects? (b) Do these side effects advance shared political values, and, if so, how? And (c) Do these side effects hinder shared political values and/or advance controversial non-political values and, if so, how?* It is important to stress here that this question is different from questions (1) and (2). Those focused on the intended aims of the policy, whereas question (3) focuses on its unintended (but often foreseeable) side effects which, we stressed in Chapter 6, may sometimes impose excessive burdens on certain individuals and groups.

The first step here is to identify any unintended positive and, especially, negative effects of the policy. These may be health effects and other, non-health effects (e.g. social, psychological, and economic effects). In some cases, these effects may be foreseeable and (almost) certain. For example, suppose that the policy under consideration is a ban on the sale of sugary drinks larger than 16 ounces in restaurants, grocery stores, and other food retail locations within a certain jurisdiction (such as the soda ban proposed by NYC in 2012). It is foreseeable, in fact certain, that this ban would limit the products that food companies and food retailers can sell in that jurisdiction. It is also certain that the ban would reduce consumers' choice of beverage products: larger sugary drinks would no longer be sold, and thus consumers would no longer be able to purchase them. If one believes that curtailing individual liberties is pro tanto undesirable from a liberal perspective, then this is a foreseeable and certain negative effect of the policy.

In other cases, the effects of a policy may be uncertain and initially unknown. For example, suppose that the policy under consideration is a program that encourages parents to make home-cooked dinners several nights each week. When the policy is first conceived, it may be uncertain whether it will have any negative effects. However, policymakers should make an effort to foresee these effects, by drawing on existing empirical evidence. If the latter is not available or is insufficient, policymakers should consider commissioning more research. Policymakers should also consider creating mechanisms of consultation through which citizens and/or communities may raise concerns regarding the potential negative effects of the policy for them. This consultation could involve probing the role served by the food or eating behaviour in question in the context of people's lives and life plans as well as the likely effects of the policy in question on them. For example, by considering relevant research (Bowen et al. 2014) and by consulting with the relevant citizens and communities, those designing the programme promoting home-cooking amongst parents may conclude that it is likely (but not certain) that this intervention will significantly increase the time women spend cooking and doing other feeding work (e.g. shopping, meal planning, cleaning up), and that this behavioural change will be unfeasible for many low-income parents because they have little control over their work schedule.

For each of the potential positive and/or negative side effects of a policy, policymakers should then assess to what extent these promote or hinder shared political values. They should do this by asking questions such as (but not limited) to the following:

- How likely is it that these side effects will promote or hinder some people's exercise of their basic rights and liberties?
- How likely is it that these side effects will promote or hinder equality of opportunity, people's individual well-being and their ability to form and enact their life plan, and/or the common good?
- How likely is it that these side effects will either remedy or exacerbate existing forms of injustice? These could include, but are not limited to, unjust inequalities based on gender, race/ethnicity, socio-economic status, or cultural or religious background, as well as the marginalization or exclusion of certain groups from key areas of public life. The inequalities in question might concern health, economics, social standing and respect, and political participation, amongst other areas.
- How likely is it that these side effects will make it particularly burdensome for members of certain groups to pursue their culturally significant food experiences?[2]

---

[2] Here we draw on Jonathan Quong's (2006) view that 'laws that force cultural or religious minorities to choose between their beliefs and basic civic opportunities represent a denial of fair equality

For example, when considering the behavioural intervention that promotes home-cooking amongst parents, one might conclude that because this intervention is likely to exacerbate existing gender inequalities in domestic work, it hinders the shared political value of gender equality. One might also conclude that because the behavioural change is infeasible for low-income parents, it will exacerbate income-based health inequalities.

When evidence shows that a policy does impose excessive negative effects ('strains of commitment') on certain individuals or groups, policymakers should consider modifying it in such a way that those effects are eliminated or significantly reduced.

In some cases, there may be disagreement about whether a particular side effect implicates particular political values or not. For example, consider the reduction in consumer choice caused by banning the sale of large sugary drinks. Some people may think that having consumer choice that is unfettered by government regulation is a basic and important liberty, and thus the ban undermines a basic liberty. Others may think that having unfettered consumer choice, i.e. having access to whatever product someone might wish to sell, is not a basic and important liberty; markets and the products sold in them are pervasively constructed and shaped by government regulation and are not properly understood as sites of free exchange that it is problematic for the government to interfere with.

This part of the framework (question 3) is essentially where a broad set of ethical objections to policies can get lodged: the potential negative effects of policies get registered, and there is consideration about whether and in what way these effects are objectionable. What is distinctive about our framework, as compared to other frameworks, is that the objections lodged get assessed based on a public reason criterion: do these objections actually implicate political values, or, on the contrary, are only controversial non-political values at stake? When considering whether the effects of

of opportunity' (p. 63). More specifically, Quong argues, '[f]air equality of opportunity should ... be construed in the wider sense — looking at each individual's complete set of primary opportunities. If the basic structure of society is organised in a way that enables one person to take advantage of all the primary opportunities in life (employment, education, family life, culture, religion), but forces another person to make zero-sum choices between these opportunities, then we should say that this basic structure does not realise the principle of fair equality of opportunity' (pp. 68–69). Hence, healthy eating efforts that force members of certain groups to choose, say, between health and employment opportunities, on the one hand, and culture and family life, on the other hand, are unreasonable from a public reason perspective.

policies are objectionable (i.e. whether they hinder political values), it may be helpful to consult the ethics literature and other academic literatures that explicitly address these issues.

7.4.4 Does the policy strike a reasonable balance of political values?

The fourth and final question is (4) *Does the policy strike a reasonable balance of political values?* Policymakers should consider whether the full set of political values relevant to the policy has been considered and whether the balance between them is reasonable: has any political value been neglected or overly de-prioritized compared to others? In answering this question, policymakers should consider again how likely it is that the policy will realize its main intended aims/political values as well as the extent to which any of its positive or negative side effects are likely to promote or hinder (other) political values. If it proves difficult to justify the policy based on a reasonable balance of political values, policymakers should repeal it or modify it in such a way that it meets this desideratum.

This is the step of the framework where the 'balancing' of values occurs. Even if the policy has some strikes against it (i.e. it hinders some political values), it may still be justifiable because of the ways in which it helps to realize other political values. For example, suppose that the behavioural intervention promoting home-cooking amongst parents was shown to be very effective amongst a subset of lower-middle-income families in improving the diet of their children, and thereby in advancing certain important political values vis-à-vis them (e.g. equality of opportunity, health equity, etc.). Suppose also that it is a cost-effective intervention. Even though the policy is also likely to exacerbate existing gender inequalities (and thus hinder gender equality) and to exacerbate health inequity vis-à-vis low-income (as opposed to lower-middle-income) parents, it could still be judged to strike a reasonable balance of political values. This may especially be the case if the policy could be paired with another policy that specifically targets low-income families—and thus advances health equity vis-à-vis them—and a policy that addresses gender inequalities.

We should expect that different people may reach different conclusions about whether a policy strikes a reasonable balance of political values (just as they might reach different conclusions about whether an effect of the policy implicates a political value to begin with). It is important for policymakers (or for whoever is using the framework) to consider how others might disagree with their conclusions about the policy. In order to prompt this kind of reflection, the framework has another key feature. When addressing each of the four questions, policymakers (or whoever is using the framework) should consider (i) how they (or other kinds of professionals, experts, or advocates) would answer the question; (ii) how a typical member of the public/community (or communities) targeted or affected by the policy would answer it (and, if there are several relevant distinct groups, how a typical member of each of them would answer it); (iii) how someone with a worldview or ideology different from theirs (and, more generally, from the view[s] that is/are dominant amongst policymakers) would answer it; and (iv) if there is disagreement amongst these three answers to the question, how a fair-minded group of people who are listening to everyone's point of view, but also trying to reach agreement, would resolve this issue. The purpose of this exercise is to simulate actual public reasoning and deliberation by asking the framework user(s) (e.g. a public health official) to realize that their normative perspective is one amongst many, not the only nor the best one. Educating the user(s) to engage in counterfactual reasoning that considers potential alternative perspectives on an issue or policy can help them to question their own assumptions and to advance public justification and public reason.

7.5. An institutionalized approach

In developing our ethics framework for public justification, we have so far considered public reasoning only by individual policymakers. However, public reasoning is perhaps best realized via more institutionalized approaches which build norms of public reason into political institutions and processes. It is therefore important to include collective institutionalized bodies in the process of public reasoning, alongside the forms of public reasoning that should be undertaken by government agencies (i.e. health departments) and legislatures.

In view of these considerations, governments should make greater use of consultation and deliberative democracy institutions in the design of healthy eating efforts. Deliberative democracy, we saw in Chapter 2, aims at ensuring procedural fairness; educating citizens to skills such as other-regardingness and respect for other people's views; helping them to better understand, articulate, and justify their own preferences and values; and, overall, contributing to more legitimate and effective policy making. The institutions that we advocate here may take various forms, including consultation by submission (i.e. citizens submit responses to consultation questions),[3] citizens' juries, consensus and citizen conferences, and local food policy councils (Ankeny 2016). These deliberation and consultation institutions are meant to advise policymaking and, in some cases, to make policy or legislation. The purpose of employing deliberation and consultation institutions is twofold. First, these institutions can help facilitate public reasoning (a central feature of deliberative democracy) amongst citizens and between policymakers and members of the public with different social backgrounds. They can do so by encouraging participants to listen to other people's opinions, learn about their experiences and the likely impact of healthy eating efforts on them, and avoid devaluing some people's experiences. Second, and relatedly, they can provide important forums for advocates speaking on behalf of disadvantaged groups, as advocates may have experience in incorporating overlooked perspectives into public discourse.[4]

Deliberation and consultation institutions can be used at all policy levels (national, international, and local) (e.g. Bächtiger et al. 2018). The local level is perhaps the most interesting and productive when it comes to healthy eating policy; designing and justifying healthy eating efforts at the local level may best ensure that these efforts are informed by the input of all the relevant parties. There may be significant variation between localities in eating practices and patterns, impediments to healthier eating rooted in local food environments, and costs and benefits of healthy eating efforts. There may also be variation between localities in public reason, i.e. variation in political values or in how political values are interpreted, and variation in views about the right balance of political values. While the public reason literature normally assumes the nation-state as its unit of analysis, one might argue that different geographical areas within nation-states may present different (specific interpretations of) political values, thus making it easier for participants

---

[3] See e.g. Australian Department of Health (2020).

[4] It is worth noting, however, that including advocates in public deliberation about healthy eating efforts may raise concerns of its own. Advocacy organizations should be carefully chosen to exclude organizations that cherry-pick evidence or present other epistemic shortcomings. Insofar as advocacy organizations are being included so that they can represent the views of a particular community (and not so that they can represent an ideological position), it is important to avoid organizations that are driven by ideological goals that do not align with the perspective of the community they claim to represent or endorse more extreme positions than that community.

to engage in public justification based on a shared vocabulary of political values. For example, while one might follow Rawls in arguing that the US public political culture presents shared political values, one might also point out that these values are interpreted and ranked differently in different US regions (e.g. rural Oklahoma vs. NYC) due to historical and cultural factors. Furthermore, the negative and positive effects of healthy eating efforts, and their implications for the realization of political values, might vary from place to place and also be more easily assessable at the local level. Therefore, it may be desirable to carry out the process of public justification at this level, as far as possible.

Moreover, healthy eating policy may be more effective when designed at the local level, because policies can be tailor-made to local needs and practices and to the local food environment. Indeed many researchers have argued for community-level and community-led design of healthy eating policy—in order to improve the effectiveness of the policies, but also to help build a coalition that will support the policies (Coughlin and Smith 2017; Huang et al. 2015; Korn et al. 2018).

Local food policy planning, which could incorporate healthy eating policy as well as other types of food policy, has been adopted in various settings— e.g. local food policy councils in the US (Blackmar 2014); the People's Food Policy Project (2011) in Canada, which emphasized the importance of food sovereignty; and the People's Food Plan in Australia (Australian Food Sovereignty Alliance 2013). As Ankeny (2016) points out, local food planning can be very inclusive towards otherwise marginalized individuals and groups. Furthermore, she claims,

> [l]ocal food planning can permit inclusion not only of 'consumers', but also [of] food producers and others involved in the food system, hence promoting future networking within communities. As with many other types of public events, local food planning often involves facilitation by those who are knowledgeable (about food policy, security, and sovereignty, for instance) but does not privilege them as experts, allowing a levelling effect that can have a positive impact on subsequent exchanges and participation, which in turn could make positive contributions at the macro level. (p. 17)

Who should be involved in consultation and deliberation processes at the local level? Alongside public health officials and ordinary citizens, there could be advocacy groups, including anti-hunger and anti-poverty groups, community organizations focused on food or agriculture (such as food justice organizations or environmental organizations), and groups that advocate for racial, ethnic, or religious minorities. Representatives of other affected local groups should also be included. These may include industry representatives, unions or labour representatives, store owners, restaurant owners, and school cafeteria workers; who exactly is included may vary depending on the policy in question. It is especially important that groups which are (or risk being) overly burdened by a policy are included in these processes and given voice.

Finally, it is important to stress that an inclusive process of deliberation and consultation in the design of healthy eating efforts can contribute to the public justification of such efforts in an additional way, i.e. by guaranteeing full (as opposed to *pro tanto*) public justification (Rawls 2005a, pp. 386–87). Full justification, we explained in Chapter 5, occurs when citizens endorse political rules based not only on public reasons but also on reasons grounded in their own conceptions of the good, which are diverse and may be non-public (e.g. a conception of the good rooted in one's religious faith). In other words, ideally citizens will endorse a policy not only because it advances shared political values that they accept as a member of their political community but also because they can see that policy as being justified from the perspective of their different conceptions of the good. If this 'overlapping consensus' of conceptions of the good can be achieved, it can also help realize a more stable liberal political order over time (Rawls 2005a, p. 65). An inclusive process of deliberation and consultation in the design of healthy eating efforts can allow different individuals and groups to better understand and explain how those efforts can be justified from the perspective of their diverse conceptions of the good.

7.6. Applying the framework:
Excluding sugary drinks from SNAP

In order to illustrate our framework and show its relevance to actual policy-making, we will use it to analyze a particular healthy eating policy: prohibiting participants in the Supplemental Nutrition Assistance Program (SNAP), the US's largest food assistance programme, from using their food assistance to purchase sugary drinks. This policy has been proposed numerous times by state-level policymakers in the US and has generated disagreement and controversy amongst ethicists, advocates, and policymakers themselves. Therefore, it may prove to be a fruitful example for illustrating our framework.

SNAP provides food support for ~40 million Americans annually, giving them an average monthly benefit of $125 to $130/person (Food and Nutrition Service, US Department of Agriculture 2019). SNAP assistance can be used to purchase virtually all food items from participating stores; only alcohol, hot prepared foods, and foods meant to be eaten in the store cannot be purchased with it (Food and Nutrition Service, US Department of Agriculture 2020). SNAP assistance also cannot be used in restaurants. According to one estimate, 9.3% of SNAP assistance is used to purchase sweetened beverages (which include sugary soft drinks, energy drinks, and sweetened tea, amongst other sweetened beverages) (O'Connor 2017). Because of the negative health effects of sugary drinks consumption, public health and other government officials have contemplated excluding sugary drinks from those foods eligible for purchase with SNAP assistance.

SNAP is administered at the state level; state agencies enrol eligible participants and distribute benefits. Policymakers in more than a dozen US states—including city mayors, officials in health departments, and legislators—have sought to exclude sugary drinks from the foods eligible for purchase with SNAP assistance (Paarlberg et al. 2018; Pomeranz and Chriqui 2015). However, states do not have the authority to do so; that authority resides at the federal level, with the US Department of Agriculture (USDA); therefore, states must petition the USDA if they wish to exclude sugary drinks from SNAP. The USDA has always denied states' requests to modify SNAP (Paarlberg et al. 2018).

Let's now consider how our framework could be used to analyse this proposed policy. As discussed earlier, ideally healthy eating policy will be designed and assessed at the local level. Accordingly, we will consider a proposed policy to exclude sugary drinks from the foods that can be purchased with SNAP in a city (let's call it City X). For simplicity, we will model this policy after an actual example. In 2010, New York State petitioned the USDA for permission to try out excluding sugary drinks from SNAP (see Barnhill 2011 for more detail). Specifically, New York State asked to conduct a demonstration project in which sugary drinks would be excluded from SNAP in NYC for a period of two years, with the effects of the exclusion being monitored and evaluated. The policy applied to sweetened beverages with more than 10 calories per cup, excluding fruit juice without added sugar, milk products, and milk substitutes.

How could our framework be used to analyse this proposed policy, and who should be involved in analysing it? As discussed earlier, ideally the policy would be analysed at the local level and by a group of stakeholders that represents various interests and perspectives on the policy. This would include public health officials in City X who are considering the policy. It would also include those most affected by the policy—in this case, participants in the food assistance programme who live in City X. According to a survey by Long et al. (2014), 54% of SNAP participants, surveyed in 2012, would support excluding sugary drinks from SNAP; given this evidence that SNAP participants are divided on this policy, it would be important to include SNAP participants who support the policy as well as those who oppose it.

Advocates should also be involved. These include representatives from anti-hunger and anti-poverty advocacy groups, which have generally been opposed to SNAP exclusions. Advocates who support SNAP exclusions should also be included. Furthermore, representatives from groups that advocate for racial/ethnic minorities should also be included, if they take a position on the policy. For example, the NAACP and the Hispanic Federation (2012) have previously advocated against policies targeting sugary drinks; if they have a stated position on this policy, they should be included, or at least their views should be represented.[5]

Ideally, this group of people with different perspectives on the policy would meet and analyse the policy, working through the framework step by step and deliberating about the policy together. Since we are not able to replicate that kind of discussion in full here, we will instead suggest some examples of responses that members of this group of deliberators might provide. When there is disagreement in the responses, we will also consider how a fair-minded group of people who are listening to everyone's point of view, but also trying to reach agreement, would resolve this issue; this is meant to replicate the process of deliberation that the group would engage in. Thus, we will go through the framework question by question and note responses that might be offered by each of the following:

---

[5] Those who have economic interests at stake should also be included or at least have their views represented. These would include the soda industry, food retailers who may lose sales and revenue, and other members of the sugary drinks supply chain (e.g. those who transport the beverages) who might also suffer economic losses. For the sake of space, we have not included these perspectives in this short analysis.

- Local public health official who is considering the policy
- SNAP participant who supports the policy
- SNAP participant who opposes the policy
- Anti-hunger and anti-poverty advocate who opposes the policy
- Advocate who supports the policy
- Fair-minded group of people trying to reach agreement

Our sample responses are informed by the actual debate about this policy that has occurred in the US, the ethics literature discussing the policy, as well as our own speculation and analysis.

7.6.1 What are the public health-related aims of the sugary drink exclusion?

The local public health official identifies the public health–related aim of the policy as reducing consumption of sugary drinks by SNAP participants and thereby improving their nutrition and health (Barnhill 2011; Lynch and Bassler 2014; Ross and MacKay 2017). The public health official also identifies a secondary public health aim of the policy. They argue that excluding sugary drinks from a government food assistance programme would send a clear message that sugary drinks are bad for health (Barnhill and King 2013), which would amplify the city's and state's other efforts to educate the public about the negative health effects of sugary drinks. We assume that the other deliberators will not dispute that these are the public health aims of the policy.

(1a) **How likely is it that the policy will achieve its stated public health–related aims?**

The local public health official acknowledges that there is no direct evidence of the effects of excluding sugary drinks from SNAP, as this policy has not previously been implemented. However, they point to evidence that that 9.3% of SNAP assistance is used to purchase sweetened beverages (O'Connor 2017); thus, it stands to reason that prohibiting the purchase of sugary drinks with SNAP assistance is likely to reduce the number of sugary drinks consumed by SNAP participants.

The public health official also presents evidence on the negative public health effects of sugary drinks (excerpted from Lynch and Bassler 2014, pp. 17–18 and The Nutrition Source 2021):

- Sugary drinks are classified as 'foods of minimal nutritional value' by the USDA.
- Half of people in the US drink sugary drinks daily. One in four people get 200+ calories from sugary drinks daily. Teens get an average 226 calories/day from sugary drinks (including soda, energy drinks, sports drinks, etc.).
- Sugar-sweetened beverages are currently the largest source of added sugar in the US diet. Sweetened beverages make up 51% of added sugars consumed by Americans.
- The average American consumes 22 teaspoons (tsp) of sugar daily, whereas the American Heart Association's recommendations for maximum intake of added sugars are 9 tsp for adult men, 6 tsp for adult women, 8 tsp for teens, and 3 tsp for children.
- Excessive sugar consumption has been linked to many health problems, including obesity, type 2 diabetes, cardiovascular disease, hypertension, gout, poor diet quality, kidney damage, cancer, sleep disturbances, and oral health problems.
- Sugary drink consumption is linked in long-term studies to greater weight gain, heart disease, and diabetes. Some studies show that reducing sugary drink consumption reduces weight gain. Randomized clinical trials show that substitution of caloric beverages with non-caloric beverages or plain water will help lower weight amongst adults and adult obese women, reduce chances of developing type 2 diabetes amongst middle-aged women, and result in better weight control amongst adolescents.

Thus, the local public health official concludes that it is likely that excluding sugary drinks from SNAP would reduce sugary drinks consumption, and that such a reduction would generally result in lower sugar consumption, healthier dietary patterns, and reduced risk of weight gain, obesity, and type 2 diabetes for SNAP participants.

The anti-hunger and anti-poverty advocate who opposes the policy objects to this conclusion. They argue that excluding sugary drinks from SNAP may not actually reduce sugary drink consumption: many SNAP participants pay for food using a combination of SNAP assistance and other funds, and thus

SNAP participants could simply use their other, non-SNAP funds to purchase sugary drinks (USDA 2007). This would undermine the effectiveness of the policy, and furthermore, it could be harmful to SNAP participants, as the money they would start spending on sugary drinks may be money they need to meet their other needs.

The SNAP participant who supports the policy replies that, for them, excluding sugary drinks from SNAP *would* reduce their purchases of sugary drinks, as they would not choose to spend other funds on sugary drinks. However, they also claim that SNAP participants are likely to differ on this matter. The public health official responds that the advocates' concerns about the effectiveness of the policy are concerns that the proposed policy—which is a two-year demonstration project—is meant to assess. They cite the work of public health experts Pomeranz and Chriqui (2015, p. 430), who note that the 'very purpose of a pilot program would be to empirically test and study' assumptions, such as the assumption that SNAP participants' sugary drink consumption would not drop because they would use other funds to buy sugary drinks.

What would a fair-minded group of people trying to reach agreement about this issue conclude? Plausibly, they would argue that there is not conclusive evidence that the policy would improve the health of SNAP participants, but that it is plausible that the policy could be effective. Thus they might conclude that it is reasonable to implement the two-year demonstration project in order to obtain better evidence.

Next, let's consider the secondary public health aim of the policy: sending a clear message that sugary drinks are bad for health and thereby amplifying the city's and state's other efforts to educate the public about the negative health effects of sugary drinks. A few participants note that this message had not occurred to them, and thus it is questionable whether the public would interpret the policy in that way. The advocate who opposes the policy contends that rather than sending a message about sugary drinks, the policy sends another kind of message entirely: it sends the message that SNAP participants cannot be trusted to make good choices for themselves and therefore the government has to restrict their choices. At this point, any relevant research should be consulted, such as research on the effects of past food bans or other product bans on public attitudes. In the absence of relevant research, what would a fair-minded group of people trying to reach agreement about this issue conclude? Plausibly, they would conclude that it is unknown how exactly the public will interpret the policy, that different segments of the population will likely interpret it differently, and that public understanding of the policy and its meanings may change over time. Given the high level of uncertainty, we cannot conclude that the policy will accomplish this secondary aim.

(1b) If the policy achieves its aims, will this advance political values, and, if so, which ones?

The local public health official argues that if the policy improved the health of SNAP participants, it would in that way increase their well-being and enable them to enjoy more fully their basic rights and liberties as well as providing them with more opportunities in life (e.g. job-related ones). They also argue that improving SNAP participants' health promotes the common good, as SNAP participants comprise a significant proportion of the overall population, and promoting the public's health promotes the common good (e.g. by helping reduce healthcare costs or costs resulting from lower productivity amongst employees with diet-related illness). Some other participants object that we cannot assume that the policy would improve SNAP participants' well-being overall, even if it improves their health; if the policy has negative effects on SNAP participants, it may decrease their well-being overall, reduce their ability to enjoy basic rights and liberties, and impose upon them 'strains of commitment' that are unreasonable.

The advocate who supports the policy points out that SNAP participants are a low-income population, and people of colour are over-represented among low-income people as a result of structural racism. This advocate argues that improving SNAP participants' health advances equality of opportunity vis-à-vis them, and thus makes progress on remedying the unjust lack of equal opportunity they experience as low-income people of colour. Improving their health can also help overcome or reduce racial inequities in health outcomes, advancing justice in another important respect. Other participants do not dispute this characterization of how the policy advances political values, were the policy to achieve its primary health-related aims.

If the policy succeeded in amplifying other efforts to educate the public about the negative health effects of sugary drinks, plausibly this would promote public health, albeit indirectly and perhaps only marginally. The group agrees that when public health is improved, this advances shared political values, such as increasing citizens' enjoyment of their rights and liberties, promoting the common good, and ensuring equality of opportunity.

7.6.2 Does the sugary drink exclusion have other aims?

In this step, the non-health aims of the policy are identified and assessed. This assessment includes evaluating the likelihood of achieving these aims. Then a judgement is made about whether these aims advance or hinder shared political values and whether they advance controversial non-political values. Two non-health aims of the SNAP exclusion policy are identified.

First, the advocate who supports the policy argues that SNAP participants spend billions of dollars on sugary drinks each year, and this amounts to a massive government subsidy of the soda industry; because the soda industry is an unethical industry, the advocate argues, the government should not subsidize it in this way (O'Connor 2017).

(2a) **How likely is it that the policy will achieve this aim?**

- The advocate cites research that found that carbonated soft drinks accounted for 6.19% of the grocery bills of food-stamp users at one large supermarket chain; assuming that this figure is representative, this would translate into $4 billion of SNAP funds being spent on carbonated drinks each year, de facto 'subsidizing' the soda industry. Others point out that 'carbonated soft drinks' is a different category of beverage than 'sugary drinks', so this figure has unclear relevance (Shenkin and Jacobson 2010). However, the public health official notes that there are government data showing that 9.3% of SNAP funds are used for sweetened beverages. Thus there is good evidence that sugary drinks *are* a significant SNAP expenditure.

(2b) **Do these other aims advance shared political values, and, if so, how?**

(2c) **Do these other aims hinder shared political values and/or advance controversial non-political values, and, if so, how?**

- Some group members question whether this aim advances political values or not. The advocate's argument is based upon the view that the soda industry is an unethical industry. Some group members reject this view, arguing that the soda industry is just one amongst many legitimate economic actors in the marketplace. They also argue that many people in the broader political community would also reject this view. In the face of this disagreement amongst group members, what would a fair-minded group of people conclude? Plausibly, they would conclude that this aim does not implicate a shared political value. More specifically, they would point out that many government policies have the effect of benefitting some economic actors more than others, and that it is neither practically possible nor morally required, from the perspective of public reason, to eliminate these differential effects. They would also reassert the point that there is reasonable disagreement regarding the ethics of the soda industry's conduct, and that therefore it would not be legitimate to implement the proposed policy on the basis of a contested view of that industry.

A second non-health aim of the policy is also identified. The public health official argues that excluding sugary drinks would make SNAP a more efficient programme. The aims of SNAP include improving the nutrition and health of participants; sugary drinks do not have any nutritional value, and merely provide excess sugar and calories, which worsen the overall nutritional profile of SNAP participants' diets. Thus, excluding sugary drinks will make the programme more effective at accomplishing its aims. Also, sugary drinks are a significant programme expenditure, as already established. Since funding sugary drinks does not contribute to the programme's aims, this expenditure amounts to a significant inefficiency in the programme, the public health official argues.

(2a) How likely is it that the policy will achieve this aim?

- The advocate who opposes the policy notes that it is uncertain whether excluding sugary drinks from SNAP would make the programme more efficient. If sugary drinks are excluded from SNAP, what will participants purchase instead? If they purchase other foods with little nutritional value (e.g. candy), then these expenditures will be just as or nearly as inefficient as sugary drink expenditures. At this point, any relevant research should be consulted. For example, did past studies on sugary drinks gather data on what foods are substituted for sugary drinks when people reduce consumption of the latter? The health department might also consider doing research of their own and surveying SNAP participants in City X. In the meantime, what would a fair-minded group of people trying to reach agreement about this issue conclude? Plausibly, they would conclude that in the absence of good data about how SNAP participants' purchases will change, we cannot assume that excluding sugary drinks from SNAP will make the programme more efficient.

(2b Do these other aims advance shared political values, and, if so, how?

(2c) Do these other aims hinder shared political values and/or advance controversial non-political values, and, if so, how?

- The group agrees that if the policy did make SNAP more efficient, this would advance political values. When government programmes are made more efficient, this in a general way promotes the common good. For example, it frees up resources that may be used on other government programmes that advance other political values.

7.6.3 Is the sugary drink exclusion likely to have unintended effects?

7.6.3.1 First side effect

This is the step in the analysis where negative side effects and various ethical objections to the policy can be registered and then assessed. This assessment involves evaluating the evidence that a potential side effect will occur. It also involves assessing to what extent a side effect promotes or hinders political values and/or imposes unreasonable 'strains of commitment' on certain individuals and groups. To do that, one needs to ask questions such as (but not limited to) the following: How likely is it that these side effects will undermine some people's exercise of their basic rights and liberties? How likely is it that these side effects will advance or undermine people's individual well-being and their exercise of the second moral power, or the common good? How likely is it that these side effects will either remedy or exacerbate forms of unjust inequality (e.g. inequality of opportunity) or other forms of injustice? These could include, but are not limited to, inequalities based on gender, race/ethnicity, socio-economic status, or cultural or religious background, as well as the marginalization or exclusion of certain groups from key areas of public life. The inequalities in question could concern health, economics, social standing and respect, and political participation, amongst other types.

The advocate and SNAP participant who oppose the policy may raise four objections to it (this discussion reflects actual objections raised to SNAP exclusions).

First, the advocate may raise the concern that the policy could be embarrassing and stigmatizing, and this could have negative downstream effects on some SNAP participants (Barnhill 2011). SNAP participants who do not know about the new exclusion of sugary drinks would attempt to purchase them using SNAP assistance, would be told at the cash register that they cannot purchase them, and would thereby be revealed to other shoppers to be using SNAP assistance, which participants will find embarrassing and stigmatizing. This embarrassment, in the USDA's words, 'has the potential to stigmatize participants by singling them out as food stamp participants, and may discourage some eligible low-income persons from participating in the program' (Food and Nutrition Service, USDA 2007). Given that SNAP participation benefits participants by increasing their food security and income, any measures that discourage participation will be harmful to the population of eligible non-participants, the advocate argues.

(3a)   How likely is it that the policy will have this side effect?

The group tries to assess this concern by turning to relevant empirical evidence (Barnhill 2011). A significant percentage of people who are eligible for SNAP assistance do not use it; 14% of eligible non-participants have identified stigma as one reason why they do not enroll in the programme. But will excluding new foods from SNAP contribute significantly to that stigma? There are already some food items not eligible for purchase with SNAP participants, and other items (e.g. paper goods) that are commonly purchased in stores are also not covered by SNAP. Thus participants must already monitor what they purchase or use both SNAP assistance and other funds when they check out. Will excluding an additional category of foods cause embarrassment and stigma for SNAP participants; i.e. will it cause any more embarrassment than they might already experience, and will that deter them from using SNAP assistance in the future? These are empirical issues; the group judges that there is not sufficient empirical evidence to judge the issue either way. Those in the group opposed to the policy argue that this is not a risk worth taking; those in the group advocating for the policy argue that this is precisely the kind of issue that would be assessed through the proposed demonstration project. What would a fair-minded group of people conclude about this issue? Plausibly, they would conclude that the mere possibility that new exclusions might cause (more) embarrassment amongst SNAP participants is not a good enough reason to reject them; studying this issue is a more reasonable solution. They conclude that, if possible, the local health department should do research with SNAP participants in City X, to try and figure out whether it is possible to adequately inform them about new SNAP exclusions in order to avoid embarrassment at the checkout and to figure out whether that experience of embarrassment would be a significant deterrent to SNAP participation.

(3b) Does this side effect advance shared political values, and, if so, how?

(3c) Does this side effects hinder shared political values and/or advance controversial non-political values, and, if so, how?

The group agrees that political values are at stake. SNAP's aims of relieving poverty, reducing food insecurity, and improving the health and nutrition of low-income people advance multiple shared political values, including promoting equality of opportunity, enabling these people to enjoy more fully their basic rights and liberties, correcting income-based and race-based injustices, and promoting the common good. If the sugary drink exclusion policy were to reduce SNAP participation rates, and thereby undermine the programme's effectiveness at accomplishing its aims, this would hinder those political values. Furthermore, by causing stigma and embarrassment amongst SNAP participants the policy could potentially undermine their self-respect, which, we have seen, is also a shared political value in liberal democracies.

7.6.3.2 Second side effect

The advocate raises a second objection to the policy: the policy micromanages the choices of low-income people, singling them out for a kind of control that is not applied to other citizens. In their view, this is disrespectful and demeaning.[6] Furthermore, they assert that this treatment is rooted in disrespectful beliefs about low-income people. The advocate cites the Food Research and Action Center (2013), a leading anti-hunger advocacy group, which has written:

---

[6] For more discussion, see Barnhill and King (2013) and Schwartz (2017).

Too often such 'singling out' of the poor emanates from a frustration about the inability to deal with the problem more broadly. And too often it emanates from a stereotypical belief that the culture or behavior among the poor is different and dysfunctional . . . Avoiding singling out poor people based on misconceptions or exaggerations is just one reason restricting SNAP is the wrong path'.

The advocate points out that these beliefs about and attitudes towards low-income people—i.e. that their behaviour is caused by a dysfunctional 'culture of poverty' and thus the state is entitled to micromanage their choices—are inextricable from the racist attitude that a dysfunctional 'culture of poverty' is prevalent in some communities of colour. Along with reflecting these beliefs, the advocate argues, the policy reinforces them.

(3a) How likely is it that the policy will have this side effect?

The group considers whether there is evidence for the claims made by the advocate. Is it true that the proposed policy is motivated by beliefs about low-income people and communities of colour and their dysfunctional behaviours? Some members of the group suggest that public health policymakers are not motivated by beliefs about SNAP participants in particular, but are just targeting SNAP participants opportunistically: it is legally and politically feasible to limit sugary drink purchases with SNAP assistance, but it would not be feasible to limit sugary drink purchases by the population as a whole. These group members argue that many public health policymakers would like to reduce sugary drink consumption in the population as a whole; thus, we need not interpret the SNAP policy as rooted in negative beliefs about low-income people or communities of colour. How could this disagreement be informed by evidence and assessed? First of all, it would be necessary to check whether there is any evidence supporting the claim that public health policymakers would indeed like to reduce sugary drink consumption in the population as a whole. This evidence could be in the form of interviews with such policymakers, either in the media or in the work of social scientists. But even if this evidence was available, it might not tell us for sure whether public health policymakers hold negative beliefs about low-income people or communities of colour. That is, at least some policymakers may *both* like to reduce sugary drink consumption in the population as a whole (for health reasons) *and* hold negative beliefs about low-income people or communities of colour that motivate this policy. Whether or not public health policymakers hold these kinds of negative beliefs, and whether or not the policy is motivated in part by such beliefs, the concern remains that part of the public holds such beliefs and these will be reinforced by the policy. To assess this claim, there may be relevant qualitative research on public attitudes towards participants in social support programmes (i.e. does the public see them as having a dysfunctional 'culture of poverty'?) and research on how public attitudes are (or are not) affected by the specific design and structure of social support programmes (i.e. does eliminating choice in a programme reinforce the belief that participants cannot make good choices?). It may not be possible to ascertain with any degree of confidence how a single change to a single policy will or will not affect public attitudes towards low-income people and communities of colour.

(3b) Does this side effect advance shared political values, and, if so, how?

(3c) Does this side effect hinder shared political values and/or advance controversial non-political values, and, if so, how?

Assuming that the policy does reflect and reinforce beliefs that low-income people and/or communities of colour have a dysfunctional 'culture of poverty', does this implicate shared political values? The group agrees that this would hinder shared political values by reinforcing race-based and class-based social injustice. The group also considers the advocate's claim that the policy singles out SNAP participants and subjects them to a form of control that other citizens are not subjected to. Does this implicate shared political values? The advocate argues that this is demeaning and disrespectful. Some of the other deliberators agree, and think that the policy undermines an important form of social equality (i.e. equal respect) that *is* a shared political value: all citizens should enjoy the same self-respect, i.e. each of them should enjoy 'a . . . sense of his own value, his secure conviction that his conception of his good, his plan of life, is worth carrying out . . . [as well as] a confidence in one's ability, so far as it is within one's power, to fulfill one's intentions' (Rawls 1999, p. 386). When SNAP participants but not others are singled out for control over their food choices, this is failing to treat them with equal respect and may undermine their self-respect. Other deliberators disagree with this conclusion. They argue that having your food choices shaped by government policy is not a failure of respect; thus, there is no failure of equal respect here. In the face of this disagreement, what might a fair-minded group of people trying to reach agreement conclude? We think it would be reasonable for them to agree with either side of this disagreement.

7.6.3.3 Third side effect

The SNAP participant who is opposed to the policy raises an objection centred on consumer choice and preferences: if sugary drinks are excluded from SNAP, participants will no longer be able to purchase them. This will have a negative effect on their family, as sugary drinks are an inexpensive treat that their children enjoy and that SNAP enables them to provide to their children (cf. Fielding-Singh 2017, 2018; Paarlberg et al. 2018, p. 312). Substituting sugary drinks with water will not have the same value. The SNAP participant who supports the policy has a different perspective on it: they support excluding sugary drinks from SNAP because this would give participants an airtight reason not to purchase sugary drinks and to stop being pestered by their children.

(3a) How likely is it that the policy will have this side effect?

At this point, any relevant research on the experiences and attitudes of SNAP participants in general should be consulted. For example, according to a survey by Long et al. (2014), 54% of SNAP participants, surveyed in 2012, would support excluding sugary drinks from SNAP. Another survey found that 68% of SNAP participants would support excluding sugary drinks from SNAP if the exclusion was paired with providing additional money for healthy foods (Leung et al. 2017). Also, if it is feasible, the health department could conduct research in City X to assess how SNAP participants would be affected by the sugary drink exclusion and their attitudes about it. Would they support it? Would it have negative or positive effects on their children's dietary patterns and their relationships with their children?

(3b) Does this side effect advance shared political values, and, if so, how?

(3c) Does this side effect hinder shared political values and/or advance controversial non-political values, and, if so, how?

The group agrees that if the policy does have negative effects on family relationships, this is a real way in which the well-being of SNAP participants is diminished, and this implicates the shared political values of promoting individual well-being and their exercise of the second moral power. Similarly, if people are not able to drink the beverages that they prefer and enjoy, this is a way in which their individual well-being, and their ability to form and enact a life plan, are undermined.

7.6.3.4 Fourth side effect
The SNAP participant who opposes the policy raises a final objection to it. The exclusion of sugary drinks from SNAP is a reduction in participants' consumer choice, as they will no longer be able to afford to buy sugary drinks. In their mind, this amounts to the government taking away an important form of freedom.

(3a) How likely is it that the policy will have this side effect?

If sugary drinks are excluded from SNAP, this is likely to prevent some SNAP participants from purchasing them. As already discussed, however, it is unknown how many SNAP participants would be able to purchase sugary drinks using other funds. For those SNAP participants who are prevented from purchasing sugary drinks, this is a reduction in consumer choice.

(3b) Does this side effect advance shared political values, and, if so, how?

(3c) Does this side effect hinder shared political values and/or advance controversial non-political values, and, if so, how?

The group considers whether this reduction in consumer choice amounts to the loss of an important form of freedom. Some group members argue that in a highly consumerist society such as the US, people's actions as consumers are a fundamental form of social interaction and personal expression, and limiting their consumer choices is a restriction of an important form of freedom; this hinders the shared political value of personal freedom for them *qua* consumers. Other group members have a different perspective. They acknowledge that shared political values in the US do require rigorous protection of basic rights and liberties, but that unfettered choice of beverage is not one of these basic liberties. Restrictions on consumer choice are commonplace: a range of regulations shape and restrict the products that can be sold in order to protect consumer health and safety. Preventing consumers from purchasing all the beverages they might like to purchase is not a troubling restriction of personal freedom, much less a violation of a basic liberty. In the face of this disagreement, what might a fair-minded group of people trying to reach agreement conclude? We think it would be reasonable for them to conclude either that this policy does not hinder shared political values, or that it does hinder the shared political value of personal freedom, though only to a minimal extent. It is worth noting that this is the kind of judgement that may vary from community to community, depending upon the shared political values in a particular community.

7.6.4 Does the sugary drink exclusion strike a reasonable balance of political values?

In this last step, an overall judgement about the policy is made. This involves taking into account all the political values at stake, how these values may be advanced or hindered, what the likelihood is that this will occur, and then considering whether there is a reasonable balance of political values.

If the policy were to succeed in reducing sugary drink consumption, there is some high-quality evidence that this would reduce health risks. However, it is uncertain whether the policy would succeed in reducing sugary drink consumption; in this respect, the policy is essentially an experiment. The group concludes that whether it is justifiable to undertake this experiment depends upon the upsides and downsides of the experiment: if there are significant risks or certain harms resulting from the policy, then undertaking it is less justifiable.

First, the upsides. If the policy succeeded in improving the health of SNAP participants, this would advance a range of political values, most notably enhancing people's enjoyment of their basic rights and liberties, promoting the common good, promoting equality of opportunity, and thus making progress on remedying the unjust lack of equal opportunity that some people (including a disproportionate number of people of colour) experience as low-income people. Improving the health of low-income people and people of colour can also help make progress on social and racial inequities in health outcomes, advancing justice in another important respect. It is unclear whether the policy would increase the well-being of SNAP participants, even if it succeeded in reducing their sugary drink consumption; this depends upon whether and the extent to which the policy has negative effects on them.

Next, the downsides of the policy. It is a modest restriction of consumer choice, which this group judges does not amount to a significant restriction of personal freedom. The primary downsides of the policy concern equality and equal respect. First, there is the concern that the policy reflects and reinforces negative beliefs about and attitudes towards low-income people and communities of colour and, in so doing, reinforces race-based and class-based social injustice. Second, there is the concern that the policy singles out SNAP participants for control in a demeaning and disrespectful way. The group was divided about whether this concern implicates political values (e.g. equal respect) or not.

Given all of this, does the policy strike a reasonable balance of political values? Some of the group's participants (e.g. the public health official and the SNAP participant who supports the policy) may believe so, but some may believe that it does not. In the face of this disagreement, what would a fair-minded group of people trying to reach agreement conclude? It is plausible that it would conclude that the policy does strike a reasonable balance of political values, given the widespread agreement regarding the benefits of improving health for the advancement of key political values (if the policy is successful) and the greater disagreement and inconclusive evidence regarding the policy's negative effects. But it might also recommend that more research be conducted in order to assess whether the alleged negative effects of the policy are likely to occur, and the extent to which they may hinder the advancement of political values and impose unreasonable 'strains of commitment' upon certain groups. The process of public reasoning is an ongoing enterprise, and policies that initially appear to be publicly justified might at a later stage turn out to be unreasonable in view of further evidence and deliberation.

Conclusion

Healthy Eating Policy and Political Philosophy: Future Research Avenues

Diet-related illness is on the rise in most countries around the world. Many governments have decided to tackle this public health challenge by introducing healthy eating efforts that aim to discourage unhealthy dietary patterns. In this book, we have examined such efforts by drawing on the theoretical and conceptual resources of political philosophy, and particularly liberal political philosophy. By unpacking and applying the idea of public reason to healthy eating efforts, we have developed both a critical lens for evaluating such efforts from a philosophical perspective and a concrete ethics framework that policymakers and practitioners can employ to assess, design, or reform actual healthy eating efforts.

Central to our analysis throughout the book has been the view that the ethical issues surrounding healthy eating efforts are numerous and complex. While much public and scholarly debate has focused on issues related to paternalism and individual autonomy, there is much more at stake when policymakers design and implement healthy eating efforts. Food and eating habits, including those that pose health risks, are central to many people's life plans and conceptions of the good, and this is something that policymakers should take into account when designing healthy eating efforts. Furthermore, healthier eating patterns can impose costs and have disvalue for some people, and government efforts that try to promote such patterns should not ignore those costs or the disproportionate burdens that some individuals and groups may experience as a result of healthy eating efforts. The public reason framework that we have developed in this book aims to provide a roadmap for navigating these complex ethical challenges, and especially for balancing ethical demands that may often be in tension with each other. Yet, this is just a starting point, and we hope that this book will stimulate future work on healthy eating efforts and other areas of food policy.

Healthy Eating Policy and Political Philosophy. Anne Barnhill and Matteo Bonotti, Oxford University Press. © Oxford University Press 2022. DOI: 10.1093/oso/9780190937881.003.0009

First, while we have only surveyed key debates in political philosophy in relation to healthy eating efforts, before zooming in on the public reason lens, we believe that more work is needed in each of those areas. For example, we believe that political philosophers and public health ethicists should develop a research agenda on the idea of 'food freedom' and the implications of healthy eating efforts for different kinds of freedoms, including negative, positive, and republican conceptions. Likewise, a systematic analysis of 'food democracy', unpacking and critically evaluating what different democratic theories entail for healthy eating efforts, is also needed.

Second, while our analysis has focused on healthy eating efforts, the resources of political philosophy can and should also be employed to evaluate other areas of food policy, including policies promoting food security, food equity, and food sovereignty. Each of these policy areas will inevitably foreground different concepts and theories from political philosophy more than others. For example, while theories of justice and equality may be especially relevant to the analysis of food equity, democratic theories may be especially useful when it comes to theorizing food sovereignty.

Finally, in Chapter 7 we sketched the contours of how our public reason framework could potentially be institutionalized, by proposing forms of consultation and deliberation that could be incorporated into the policymaking process. However, more work is needed to identify ways of integrating the normative analysis of policies (such as our public reason framework) into policymaking processes. This will require closer interaction amongst political philosophers, public health ethicists, and public policy scholars in order to design effective approaches.

Ideally, the normative analysis of policies could be married with innovative methodologies for policy design and evaluation in order to create a holistic process that improves the effectiveness, justifiability, and political viability of policies. For example, two promising approaches to policy design which we can only briefly mention here are systems approaches and design thinking, which some public health researchers have already been using in obesity prevention policy in innovative ways.

Taking a *systems approach* to a problem or issue means understanding that it is part of a system with many interrelated parts, and that the system may work in surprising ways, as when intuitively compelling efforts backfire or produce unintended consequences elsewhere in the system (Stroh 2015). Systems approaches, which include qualitative and quantitative methodologies for modelling and mapping systems, can help policy designers grapple with complexity and break out of unproductive, conventional approaches to a problem. Systems approaches have been used in mathematics, engineering, the social sciences, and public health (Luke and Stamatakis 2012), and public health researchers have called for using systems approaches in designing food policies, including healthy eating and obesity interventions (Barnhill et al. 2018; IOM 2012; IOM and National Research Council 2015). An interesting area for future research may involve incorporating normative analysis (such as the public reason approach that we outline in this book) into systems approaches to healthy eating policies (Silva et al. 2018).

Design thinking is a technique for understanding users' needs and creating 'user-focused' products. It involves, among other elements, engaging with users (e.g. the targets of a healthy eating policy) to understand their needs and perspectives, prototyping many solutions to a problem, and multiple rounds of revising these solutions. Design thinking can contribute to the effectiveness and legitimacy of public health policy and increase citizens' trust in policymakers and institutions (Mintrom and Luetjens 2016). An interesting avenue for future research may involve incorporating normative analysis (including the public reason approach that we outline in this book) into design thinking methodologies, in order to create a unified process that involves engaging communities in design thinking about healthy eating efforts and normatively assessing any proposed policies.

We hope that our book will stimulate further research in each of these areas, in the spirit of truly interdisciplinary and policy-oriented scholarship.

Bibliography

Aaron, Daniel G. and Fatima C. Stanford (2021). 'Is Obesity a Manifestation of Systemic Racism? A Ten-Point Strategy for Study and Intervention', *Journal of Internal Medicine*, 290 (2): 416–20.

Aaron, Daniel G. and Michael B. Siegel (2016). 'Sponsorship of National Health Organizations by Two Major Soda Companies', *American Journal of Preventive Medicine*, 52 (1): 20–30.

Abu-Odeh, Desiree (2014). 'Fat Stigma and Public Health: A Theoretical Framework and Ethical Analysis', *Kennedy Institute of Ethics Journal*, 24 (3): 247–65.

Afshin, Ashkan, Renata Micha, Shahab Khatibzadeh, Laura A. Schmidt, and Dariush Mozaffarian (2014). 'Dietary Policies to Reduce Non-communicable Diseases'. In *The Handbook of Global Health Policy*, ed. Garrett W. Brown, Gavin Yamey, and Sarah Wamala (Chichester, UK: John Wiley & Sons), 175–93.

GBD 2017 Collaborators. (2019). 'Health Effects of Dietary Risks in 195 Countries, 1990–2017: A Systematic Analysis for the Global Burden of Disease Study 2017', *The Lancet*, 393 (10184): 1958–72.

Alkon, Alison Hope and Julian Agyeman (2011). *Cultivating Food Justice: Race, Class, and Sustainability* (Cambridge, MA: MIT Press).

Anderson, Eugene N. (2005). *Everyone Eats: Understanding Food and Culture* (New York: New York University Press).

Ankeny, Rachel (2016). 'Inviting Everyone to the Table: Strategies for More Effective and Legitimate Food Policy via Deliberative Approaches', *Journal of Social Philosophy*, 47 (1): 10–24.

Anonymous (2012a). 'A Soda Ban Too Far', *The New York Times*, 31 May. http://www.nytimes.com/2012/06/01/opinion/a-soda-ban-too-far.html.

Anonymous (2012b). 'Police Could Be Disciplined If They Fail Fitness Tests', *BBC News*, 15 March. http://www.bbc.co.uk/news/uk-17382096.

Anonymous (2012c). 'The Nanny State's Biggest Test: Should Governments Make Their Citizens Exercise More and Eat Less?', *The Economist*, 15 December. http://www.economist.com/news/special-report/21568074-should-governments-make-their-citizens-exercise-more-and-eat-less-nanny-states.

Anonymous (2014). 'US Court Rejects New York Supersize Soda Ban', *BBC News*, 26 June. http://www.bbc.co.uk/news/world-us-canada-28049973.

Aphramor, Lucy (2009). 'Disability and the Anti-obesity Offensive', *Disability & Society*, 24 (7): 897–909.

Arneson, Richard J. (1980). 'Mill versus Paternalism', *Ethics*, 90 (4): 470–89.

Arneson, Richard J. (2005). 'Joel Feinberg and the Justification of Hard Paternalism', *Legal Theory*, 11 (3): 259–84.

Arneson, Richard J. (2015). 'Equality of Opportunity'. In *The Stanford Encyclopedia of Philosophy*, ed. Edward N. Zalta. Summer ed. https://plato.stanford.edu/archives/sum2015/entries/equal-opportunity/.

Attwood, Angela S., Nicholas E. Scott-Samuel, George Stothart, and Marcus R. Munafò (2012). 'Glass Shape Influences Consumption Rate for Alcoholic Beverages', *PLoS ONE*, 7 (8): e43007.

Aubrey, Allison (2019). 'Bad Diets Are Responsible for More Deaths Than Smoking, Global Study Finds', *The Salt*, 3 April. https://www.npr.org/sections/thesalt/2019/04/03/709507504/bad-diets-are-responsible-for-more-deaths-than-smoking-glo bal-study-finds.

Audi, Robert (2011). *Democratic Authority and the Separation of Church and State* (New York: Oxford University Press).

Australian Department of Health (2020). 'Public Consultation: Food Regulation Policy Guideline', 2 February. https://consultations.health.gov.au/chronic-disease-and-food-policy-branch/copy-of-food-regulation-policy-guideline/.

Australian Food Sovereignty Alliance (2013). 'The People's Food Plan: A Common-Sense Approach to a Fair, Sustainable and Resilient Food System', Working Paper (revised), February. http://www.australianfoodsovereigntyalliance.org/wp-content/uploads/2012/11/AFSA_PFP_WorkingPaper-FINAL-15-Feb-2013.pdf.

Bächtiger, André, John S. Dryzek, Jane Mansbridge and, Mark E. Warren (eds.) (2018). *The Oxford Handbook of Deliberative Democracy* (Oxford: Oxford University Press).

Backett, Kathryn, Charlie Davison, and Kenneth Mullen (1994). 'Lay Evaluation of Health and Healthy Lifestyles: Evidence from Three Studies', *British Journal of General Practice*, 44 (383): 277–80.

Backholer, Kathryn, Adyya Gupta, Christina Zorbas, Rebecca Bennett, Oliver Huse, Alexandra Chung, Anna Isaacs, Gabby Golds, Bridget Kelly, and Anna Peeters (2021). 'Differential Exposure to, and Potential Impact of, Unhealthy Advertising to Children by Socio-economic and Ethnic Groups: A Systematic Review of the Evidence', *Obesity Reviews*, 22 (3): e13144.

Badano, Gabriele and Alasia Nuti (2018). 'Under Pressure: Political Liberalism, the Rise of Unreasonableness, and the Complexity of Containment', *The Journal of Political Philosophy*, 26 (2): 145–68.

Badano, Gabriele, and Alasia Nuti (2020). 'The Limits of Conjecture: Political Liberalism, Counter-Radicalisation and Unreasonable Religious Views.' *Ethnicities* 20 (2): 293–311.

Badano, Gabriele and Matteo Bonotti (2020). 'Rescuing Public Reason Liberalism's Accessibility Requirement', *Law and Philosophy*, 39 (1): 35–65.

Bailey, Zinzi D., Nancy Krieger, Madina Agénor, Jasmine Graves, Natalia Linos, and Mary T. Bassett (2017). 'Structural Racism and Health Inequities in the USA: Evidence and Interventions', *The Lancet*, 389 (10077): 1453–63.

Barnes, Elizabeth (1996). *The Minority Body: A Theory of Disability* (New York: Oxford University Press).

Barnhill, Anne (2011). 'Impact and Ethics of Excluding Sweetened Beverages from the SNAP Program', *American Journal of Public Health*, 101 (11): 2037–43.

Barnhill, Anne (2014). 'What Is Manipulation?' In *Manipulation*, ed. Michael Weber and Christian Coons (Oxford: Oxford University Press), 51–72.

Barnhill, Anne (2016). 'I'd Like to Teach the World to Think: Commercial Advertising and Manipulation', *Journal of Marketing Behavior*, 1 (3–4): 307–28.

Barnhill, Anne (2019). 'Obesity Prevention and Promotion of Good Nutrition: Public Health Ethics Issues'. In *The Oxford Handbook of Public Health Ethics*, ed. Anna C. Mastroianni, Jeffrey P. Kahn, and Nancy E. Kass (Oxford: Oxford University Press), 585–596.

Barnhill, Anne, Anne Palmer, Christine M. Weston, Kelly D. Brownell, Kate Clancy, Christina D. Economos, Joel Gittelsohn, Ross A. Hammond, Shiriki Kumanyika, and Wendy L. Bennett (2018). 'Grappling with Complex Food Systems to Reduce Obesity: A US Public Health Challenge', *Public Health Reports*, 133 (1suppl.): 44S–53S.

Barnhill, Anne and Katherine F. King (2013). 'Evaluating Equity Critiques in Food Policy: The Case of Sugar-Sweetened Beveragess', *The Journal of Law, Medicine & Ethics*, 41 (1): 301–9.

Barnhill, Anne, Katherine F. King, Nancy Kass, and Ruth Faden (2014). 'The Value of Unhealthy Eating and the Ethics of Healthy Eating Efforts', *Kennedy Institute of Ethics Journal*, 24 (3): 187–217.

Barry, Brian (2001). *Culture and Equality: An Egalitarian Critique of Multiculturalism.* (Cambridge, MA: Harvard University Press).

Barry, Colleen L., Jeff Niederdeppe, and Sarah E. Gollust (2013). 'Taxes on Sugar-Sweetened Beverages: Results from a 2011 National Public Opinion Survey', *American Journal of Preventive Medicine*, 44 (2): 158–63.

Bayer, Ronald (2007). 'The Continuing Tensions between Individual Rights and Public Health: Talking Point on Public Health versus Civil Liberties', *EMBO Reports*, 8 (12): 1099–103.

Bayer, Ronald (2008a). 'Stigma and the Ethics of Public Health: Not Can We but Should We', *Social Science & Medicine*, 67 (3): 463–72.

Bayer, Ronald (2008b). 'What Means This Thing Called Stigma? A Response to Burris', *Social Science & Medicine*, 67 (3): 476–77.

Bayer, Ronald and Jonathan D. Moreno (1986). 'Health Promotion: Ethical and Social Dilemmas of Government Policy', *Health Affairs*, 5 (2): 72–85.

Bayol, Stéphanie A., Biggy H. Simbi, J. A. Bertrand, and N. C. Stickland (2008). 'Offspring from Mothers Fed a "Junk Food" Diet in Pregnancy and Lactation Exhibit Exacerbated Adiposity That Is More Pronounced in Females', *The Journal of Physiology*, 586 (13): 3219–30.

Beauchamp, Dan E. (1976). 'Public Health as Social Justice', *Inquiry: A Journal of Medical Care Organization, Provision and Financing*, 13 (1): 3–14.

Beauchamp, Dan E. (1980). 'Public Health and Individual Liberty', *Annual Review of Public Health*, 1 (1): 121–36.

Beauchamp, Tom L. and James F. Childress (2019). *Principles of Biomedical Ethics*, 8th ed. (Oxford: Oxford University Press).

Beekman, Volkert and Frans W. A. Brom (2007). 'Ethical Tools to Support Systematic Public Deliberations about the Ethical Aspects of Agricultural Biotechnologies', *Journal of Agricultural and Environmental Ethics*, 20 (1): 3–12.

Beekman, Volkert, et al. (2006). 'Ethical Bio-Technology Assessment Tools for Agriculture and Food Production: Final Report Ethical Bio-TA Tools (QLG6-CT-2002-02594).' LEI, The Hague.

Béné, Christophe, Jessica Fanzo, Steven D. Prager, Harold A. Achicanoy, Brendan R. Mapes, Patricia Alvarez Toro, and Camila Bonilla Cedrez (2020). 'Global Drivers of Food System (Un)Sustainability: A Multi-Country Correlation Analysis', *PLoS ONE*, 15 (4): e0231071.

Benhabib, Seyla (1996). 'Toward a Deliberative Model of Democratic Legitimacy'. In *Democracy and Difference: Contesting the Boundaries of the Political*, ed. Seyla Benhabib (Princeton, NJ: Princeton University Press), 67–94.

Bennett, Wendy L., Renee F. Wilson, Allen Zhang, Eva Tseng, Emily A. Knapp, Hadi Kharrazi, Elizabeth A. Stuart, Oluwaseun Shogbesan, and Eric B. Bass (2018). 'Methods for Evaluating Natural Experiments in Obesity: A Systematic Review', *Annals of Internal Medicine*, 168 (11): 791–800.

Bentham, Jeremy ([1789] 1907). *An Introduction to the Principles of Morals and Legislation* (Oxford: Clarendon Press).

Berlin, Isaiah (1969). 'Two Concepts of Liberty'. In *Four Essays on Liberty* (Oxford: Oxford University Press), 118–72.

Berofsky, Bernard (1995). *Liberation from Self* (New York: Cambridge University Press).

Bhattacharya, Jay and M. Kate Bundorf (2009). 'The Incidence of the Healthcare Costs of Obesity', *Journal of Health Economics*, 28 (3): 649–58.

Binmore, Ken (2000). 'A Utilitarian Theory of Legitimacy'. In *Economics, Values, and Organization*, ed. Avner Ben-Ner and Louis G. Putterman (Cambridge: Cambridge University Press), 101–32.

Bird, Colin (2014). 'Coercion and Public Justification', *Politics, Philosophy and Economics*, 13 (3): 189–214.

Bittman, Mark (2013). 'Pollan Cooks!', *The New York Times*, 18 April. http://query.nyti mes.com/gst/fullpage.html.

Bittman, Mark (2014). 'Rethinking Our "Rights" to Dangerous Behaviors', *The New York Times*, 25 February. http://www.nytimes.com/2014/02/26/opinion/bittman-rethink ing-our-rights-to-dangerous-behaviors.html.

Black, Jane (2010). 'Small Changes Steer Kids toward Smarter School Lunch Choices', *Washington Post*, 9 June. http://www.washingtonpost.com/wp-dyn/content/article/ 2010/06/08/AR2010060800999.html.

Blackmar, Jeannette M. (2014). 'Deliberative Democracy, Civic Engagement and Food Policy Councils', *Rivista di Studi sulla Sostenibilità*, 2 (2): 43–57.

Bleich, Sara N. and Jamy D. Ard (2021). 'COVID-19, Obesity, and Structural Racism: Understanding the Past and Identifying Solutions for the Future', *Cell Metabolism*, 33 (2): 234–41.

Bleich, Sara N., Hannah G. Lawman, Michael T. LeVasseur, Jiali Yan, Nandita Mitra, Caitlin M. Lowery, Ana Peterhans, Sophia Hua, Laura A. Gibson, and Christina A. Roberto (2020). 'The Association of a Sweetened Beverage Tax with Changes in Beverage Prices and Purchases at Independent Stores', *Health Affairs*, 39 (7): 1130–39.

Bohman, James (1998). 'Survey Article: The Coming of Age of Deliberative Democracy', *The Journal of Political Philosophy*, 6 (4): 400–425.

Bohman, James and Henry S. Richardson (2009). 'Liberalism, Deliberative Democracy, and "Reasons That All Can Accept"', *The Journal of Political Philosophy*, 17 (3): 253–74.

Bonotti, Matteo (2014). 'Food Labels, Autonomy, and the Right (Not) to Know', *Kennedy Institute of Ethics Journal*, 24 (4): 301–21.

Bonotti, Matteo (2015). 'Food Policy, Nutritionism, and Public Justification', *Journal of Social Philosophy*, 46 (4): 402–17.

Bonotti, Matteo (2017). *Partisanship and Political Liberalism in Diverse Societies* (Oxford: Oxford University Press).

Bonotti, Matteo (2020a). 'Republican Food Sovereignty', *Philosophy & Social Criticism*, 46 (4): 390–411.

Bonotti, Matteo (2020b). 'Must Politics Be War? Restoring Our Trust in the Open Society. By Kevin Vallier. New York: Oxford University Press, 2019. 256p. $85.00 cloth', *Perspectives on Politics*, 18 (1): 248–49.

Bonotti, Matteo and Steve T. Zech (2021). *Recovering Civility During COVID-19* (Singapore: Palgrave Macmillan).

Bonotti, Matteo and Gideon Calder (2021). 'Health, Children's Well-Being, and Opportunity Pluralism', unpublished manuscript.

Bowen, Ronni Lee and Carol M. Devine (2011). ' "Watching a Person Who Knows How to Cook, You'll Learn a Lot": Linked Lives, Cultural Transmission, and the Food Choices of Puerto Rican Girls', *Appetite*, 56 (2): 290–98.

Bowen, Sarah, Sinikka Elliott, and Joslyn Brenton (2014). 'The Joy of Cooking?', *Contexts*, 13 (3): 20–25.

Braveman, Paula (2014). 'What Are Health Disparities and Health Equity? We Need to Be Clear', *Public Health Reports*, 129 (suppl. 2): 5–8.

Braveman, Paula A., Catherine Cubbin, Susan Egerter, David R. Williams, and Elsie Pamuk (2010). 'Socioeconomic Disparities in Health in the United States: What the Patterns Tell Us', *American Journal of Public Health*, 100 (suppl. 1): S186–S196.

Braveman, Paula and Laura Gottlieb (2014). 'The Social Determinants of Health: It's Time to Consider the Causes of the Causes', *Public Health Reports*, 129 (suppl. 2): 19–31.

Braveman, Paula A., Shiriki Kumanyika, Jonathan Fielding, Thomas LaVeist, Luisa N. Borrell, Ron Manderscheid, and Adewale Troutman (2011). 'Health Disparities and Health Equity: The Issue Is Justice', *American Journal of Public Health*, 101 (suppl. 1): S149–S155.

Bremer, Scott, Mohammad Mahfujul Haque, Arne Sveinson Haugen, and Matthias Kaiser (2016). 'Inclusive Governance of Aquaculture Value-Chains: Co-Producing Sustainability Standards for Bangladeshi Shrimp and Prawns', *Ocean & Coastal Management*, 131: 13–24.

Brennan, Jason (2018). 'A Libertarian Case for Mandatory Vaccination', *Journal of Medical Ethics*, 44 (1): 37–43.

Bridging the Gap (2014). 'Laws for School Snack Foods and Beverages Vary Widely from State to State', 21 January. http://foods.bridgingthegapresearch.org/.

Brownell, Kelly D. and Kenneth E. Warner (2009). 'The Perils of Ignoring History: Big Tobacco Played Dirty and Millions Died. How Similar Is Big Food?', *Milbank Quarterly*, 87 (1): 259–94.

Brownell, Kelly D., Rogan Kersh, David S. Ludwig, Robert C. Post, Rebecca M. Puhl, Marlene B. Schwartz, and Walter C. Willett (2010). 'Personal Responsibility and Obesity: A Constructive Approach to a Controversial Issue', *Health Affairs*, 29 (3): 379–87.

Burris, Scott (2008). 'Stigma, Ethics and Policy: A Commentary on Bayer's "Stigma and the Ethics of Public Health: Not Can We but Should We" ', *Social Science & Medicine*, 67 (3): 473–75.

Buss, Sarah (2005). 'Valuing Autonomy and Respecting Persons: Manipulation, Seduction, and the Basis of Moral Constraints', *Ethics*, 115 (2): 195–235.

Byrne, S., Z. Cooper, and C. Fairburn (2003). 'Weight Maintenance and Relapse in Obesity: A Qualitative Study', *International Journal of Obesity and Related Metabolic Disorders*, 27 (8): 955–62.

Carrington, Christopher (1999). *No Place Like Home: Relationships and Family Life among Lesbians and Gay Men* (Chicago: University of Chicago Press).

Carvalho, Teresa G. (2020). 'Donald Trump Is Taking Hydroxychloroquine to Ward Off COVID-19: Is That Wise?', *The Conversation*, 21 May. https://theconversation.com/don ald-trump-is-taking-hydroxychloroquine-to-ward-off-covid-19-is-that-wise-139031.

Cawley, John (2004). 'The Impact of Obesity on Wages', *Journal of Human Resources*, 39 (2): 451–74.

Cawley, John and Feng Liu (2012). 'Maternal Employment and Childhood Obesity: A Search for Mechanisms in Time Use Data', *Economics and Human Biology*, 10 (4): 352–64.

Center for Science in the Public Interest (2019). 'State and Local Restaurant Kids' Meal Policies', http://www.foodmarketing.org/wp-content/uploads/2019/02/local_kids_meal_policies_february_2019.pdf.

Centers for Disease Control and Prevention (2020a). 'National Diabetes Statistics Report'. https://www.cdc.gov/diabetes/pdfs/data/statistics/national-diabetes-statistics-report.pdf.

Centers for Disease Control and Prevention (2020b). 'Adult Obesity Facts'. https://www.cdc.gov/obesity/data/adult.html.

Chambers, Simone (1996). *Reasonable Democracy* (Ithaca, NY: Cornell University Press).

Chappell, Zsuzsanna (2012). *Deliberative Democracy: A Critical Introduction* (New York: Palgrave Macmillan).

Chetty, Raj, Michael Stepner, Sarah Abraham, Shelby Lin, Benjamin Scuderi, Nicholas Turner, Augustin Bergeron, and David Cutler (2016). 'The Association between Income and Life Expectancy in the United States, 2001–2014', *JAMA*, 315 (16): 1750–66.

Childress, James F., Ruth R. Faden, Ruth D. Gaare, Lawrence O. Gostin, Jeffrey Kahn, Richard J. Bonnie, Nancy E. Kass, Anna C. Mastroianni, Jonathan D. Moreno, and Phillip Nieburg (2002). 'Public Health Ethics: Mapping the Terrain', *The Journal of Law, Medicine & Ethics*, 30 (2): 170–78.

Christakis, Nicholas A. and James H. Fowler (2007). 'The Spread of Obesity in a Large Social Network over 32 Years', *New England Journal of Medicine*, 357 (4): 370–77.

Christman, John (2018). 'Autonomy in Moral and Political Philosophy'. In *The Stanford Encyclopedia of Philosophy*, ed. Edward N. Zalta. Spring ed. https://plato.stanford.edu/archives/spr2018/entries/autonomy-moral/.

Clarke, Simon (2006). 'Debate: State Paternalism, Neutrality and Perfectionism', *The Journal of Political Philosophy*, 14 (1): 111–21.

Clayton, Matthew and David Stevens (2014). 'When God Commands Disobedience: Political Liberalism and Unreasonable Religions', *Res Publica*, 20 (1): 65–84.

Cohen, Deborah and Thomas A. Farley (2008). 'Eating as an Automatic Behavior', *Preventing Chronic Disease*, 5 (1): A23.

Cohen, Gerald A. (1988). *History, Labour and Freedom: Themes from Marx* (Oxford: Clarendon Press).

Cohen, Joshua (1993). 'Freedom of Expression', *Philosophy & Public Affairs*, 22 (3): 207–63.

Cohen, Joshua (1996). 'Procedure and Substance in Deliberative Democracy'. In *Democracy and Difference: Contesting the Boundaries of the Political*, ed. Seyla Benhabib (Princeton, NJ: Princeton University Press), 95–119.

Cohen, Joshua (2010). *The Arc of the Moral Universe and Other Essays* (Cambridge, MA: Harvard University Press).

Colgrove, James and Ronald Bayer (2005). 'Manifold Restraints: Liberty, Public Health, and the Legacy of *Jacobson v Massachusetts*', *American Journal of Public Health*, 95 (4): 571–76.

Committee on World Food Security (2021). 'Voluntary Guidelines on Food Systems and Nutrition'. https://www.who.int/teams/nutrition-food-safety/cfs-voluntary-guidelines-on-food-systems-and-nutrition.

Conly, Sarah (2013a). *Against Autonomy: Justifying Coercive Paternalism* (Cambridge: Cambridge University Press).

Conly, Sarah (2013b). 'Coercive Paternalism in Health Care: Against Freedom of Choice', *Public Health Ethics*, 6 (3): 241–45.

Coons, Christian and Michael Weber (2014). *Manipulation* (Oxford: Oxford University Press).

Coughlin, Steven S. and Selina A. Smith (2017). 'Community-Based Participatory Research to Promote Healthy Diet and Nutrition and Prevent and Control Obesity among African-Americans: A Literature Review', *Journal of Racial and Ethnic Health Disparities*, 4 (2): 259–68.

Counihan, Carole and Penny Van Esterik (2013). *Food and Culture: A Reader* (New York: Routledge).

Courtwright, Andrew (2013). 'Stigmatization and Public Health Ethics', *Bioethics*, 27 (2): 74–80.

Crocker, Lawrence (1980). *Positive Liberty* (London: Nijhoff).

Cross, Ben and Thomas M. Besch (2019). 'Why Inconclusiveness Is a Problem for Public Reason', *Law and Philosophy*, 38 (4): 407–32.

Cruwys, Tegan, Kirsten E. Bevelander, and Roel C. J. Hermans (2015). 'Social Modeling of Eating: A Review of When and Why Social Influence Affects Food Intake and Choice', *Appetite*, 86: 3–18.

Dale, Daniel (2020). 'Fact Check: Trump Made at Least 22 False or Misleading Claims at ABC Town Hall', *CNN*, 16 September. https://edition.cnn.com/2020/09/16/politics/fact-check-trump-abc-town-hall/index.html.

Daniels, N. (2008). *Just Health: Meeting Health Needs Fairly* (New York: Cambridge University Press).

Davies, Lizzie (2013). 'Italy Claims "Traffic-Light" Labelling Unfair on Mediterranean Food', *The Guardian*, 22 October. https://www.theguardian.com/world/2013/oct/21/italy-traffic-light-food-labels-unfair.

Davis, Debra C., Mary C. Henderson, Anne Boothe, Merriam Douglass, Sandra Faria, Daphne Kennedy, Edeth Kitchens, and Mary Weaver (1992). 'Health Beliefs and Practices of Rural Elders', *Caring*, 11 (2): 22–28.

Dawson, Angus and Marcel Verweij (2007). 'Introduction: Ethics, Prevention, and Public Health'. In *Ethics, Prevention, and Public Health*, ed. Angus Dawson and Marcel Verweij (Oxford: Oxford University Press), 1–12.

Deblonde, M., R. de Graaff, and F. Brom (2007). 'An Ethical Toolkit for Food Companies: Reflections on Its Use', *Journal of Agricultural and Environmental Ethics*, 20 (1): 99–118.

De Marneffe, Peter (2006). 'Avoiding Paternalism', *Philosophy and Public Affairs*, 34 (1): 68–94.

Department of Health and Mental Hygiene, Board of Health (2012). *Notice of Adoption of an Amendment (§81.53) to Article 81 of The New York City Health Code*. http://www.nyc.gov/html/nycrules/downloads/rules/F-DOHMH-09-13-12-a.pdf.

De Tavernier, Johan (2012). 'Food Citizenship: Is There a Duty for Responsible Consumption?', *Journal of Agricultural and Environmental Ethics*, 25 (6): 895–907.

Devine, Carol M. and Anne Barnhill (2018). 'The Ethical and Public Health Importance of Unintended Consequences: The Case of Behavioral Weight Loss Interventions', *Public Health Ethics*, 11 (3): 356–61.

Devine, Carol M., Margaret Jastran, Jennifer A. Jabs, Elaine Wethington, Tracy J. Farrell, and Carole A. Bisogni (2006). ' "A Lot of Sacrifices": Work-Family Spillover and the Food Choice Coping Strategies of Low-Wage Employed Parents', *Social Science & Medicine*, 63 (10): 2591–603.

DiBonaventura, Marco D. and Gretchen B. Chapman (2008). 'Do Decision Biases Predict Bad Decisions? Omission Bias, Naturalness Bias, and Influenza Vaccination', *Medical Decision Making*, 28 (4): 532–39.

Dicker, Ron (2012). '"Nanny Bloomberg" Ad in New York Times Targets N.Y. Mayor's Anti-Soda Crusade', *Huffington Post*, 4 June. http://www.huffingtonpost.com/2012/06/04/ nanny-bloomberg-ad-in-new_n_1568037.html.

DiLeone, Ralph J, Jane R Taylor, and Marina R Picciotto (2012). 'The Drive to Eat: Comparisons and Distinctions between Mechanisms of Food Reward and Drug Addiction.' *Nature Neuroscience* 15 (10): 1330–35.

Dixon, Beth (2018). 'Obesity and Responsibility'. In *The Oxford Handbook of Food Ethics*, ed. Anne Barnhill, Mark Budolfson, and Tyler Doggett (New York: Oxford University Press), 614–33.

Dougherty, Geoff B., Sherita H. Golden, Alden L. Gross, Elizabeth Colantuoni, and Lorraine T. Dean (2020). 'Measuring Structural Racism and Its Association with BMI', *American Journal of Preventive Medicine*, 59 (4): 530–37.

Dworkin, Gerald (1972). 'Paternalism', *Monist*, 56 (1): 64–84.

Dworkin, Gerald (1997). 'Paternalism'. In *Mill's On Liberty: Critical Essays*, ed. Gerald Dworkin (Lanham, MD: Rowman & Littlefield), 61–82.

Dworkin, Gerald (2020). 'Paternalism'. In *The Stanford Encyclopedia of Philosophy*, ed. Edward N. Zalta, Fall ed. https://plato.stanford.edu/archives/fall2020/entries/paternalism/.

Dyzenhaus, David (1992). 'John Stuart Mill and the Harm of Pornography', *Ethics*, 102 (3): 534–51.

Eberle, Christopher (2002). *Religious Convictions in Liberal Politics* (Cambridge: Cambridge University).

Edwards, John (2010). 'West Ham Fine Benni Mccarthy over Weight Deadline: Battle of the Bulge Costs Striker £80,000', *Daily Mail*, 14 September. http://www.dailymail.co.uk/sport/football/article-1311722/West-Ham-fine-Benni-McCarthy-80k-battle-bulge--EXCLUSIVE.html.

Egger, Garry and Boyd Swinburn (1997). 'An "Ecological" Approach to the Obesity Pandemic', *BMJ*, 315 (7106): 477–80.

Eldridge, Johanna D., Carol M. Devine, Elaine Wethington, Luz Aceves, Erica Phillips-Caesar, Brian Wansink, and Mary E. Charlson (2016). 'Environmental Influences on Small Eating Behavior Change to Promote Weight Loss among Black and Hispanic Populations', *Appetite*, 96: 129–37.

Elster, Jon (1983). *Sour Grapes: Studies in the Subversion of Rationality* (Cambridge: Cambridge University Press).

Enoch, David (2015). 'Against Public Reason'. In *Oxford Studies in Political Philosophy (Volume 1)*, ed. David Sobel, Peter Vallentyne and Steven Wall (Oxford: Oxford University Press), 112–42.

Estlund, David (2008). *Democratic Authority* (Princeton, NJ: Princeton University Press).

Eyal, Nir (2016). 'Nudging and Benign Manipulation for Health'. In *Nudging Health: Health Law and Behavioral Economics*, ed. I. Glenn Cohen and Holly Fernandez Lynch (Baltimore, MD: Johns Hopkins University Press), 83–96.

Faden, Ruth (1987). 'Ethical Issues in Government Sponsored Public Health Campaigns', *Health Education Quarterly*, 14 (1): 27–37.

Faden, Ruth, Justin Bernstein, and Sirine Shebaya (2020). 'Public Health Ethics'. In *The Stanford Encyclopedia of Philosophy*, edited by Edward N. Zalta, Fall ed. https://plato.stanford.edu/archives/fall2020/entries/publichealth-ethics/.

Faden, Ruth R., Nancy E. Kass, Steven N. Goodman, Peter Pronovost, Sean Tunis, and Tom L. Beauchamp (2013). 'An Ethics Framework for a Learning Health Care System: A Departure from Traditional Research Ethics and Clinical Ethics', *Hastings Center Report*, 43 (s1): S16–S27.

Fairchild, Amy L., Ronald Bayer, and James Colgrove (2015). 'Risky Business: New York City's Experience with Fear-Based Public Health Campaigns', *Health Affairs*, 34 (5): 844–51.

Falk, Laura W., Jeffrey Sobal, Carole A. Bisogni, Margaret Connors, and Carol M. Devine (2001). 'Managing Healthy Eating: Definitions, Classifications, and Strategies', *Health Education and Behavior*, 28 (4): 425–39.

Fanzo, Jessica (2019). 'Healthy and Sustainable Diets and Food Systems: The Key to Achieving Sustainable Development Goal 2?', *Food Ethics*, 4 (2): 159–74.

Farley, Thomas A. (2015). 'The Problem with Focusing on Childhood Obesity', *The New York Times*, 18 December. http://www.nytimes.com/2015/12/18/opinion/the-problem-with-focusing-on-childhood-obesity.html.

Feinberg, Joel (1971). 'Legal Paternalism', *Canadian Journal of Philosophy*, 1 (1): 105–24.

Feinberg, Joel (1986). *Harm to Self: The Moral Limits of the Criminal Law* (New York: Oxford University Press).

Fielding-Singh, Priya (2017). 'To Understand How Families Eat, Consider What Food Means to Parents', *Work in Progress*, 14 November. https://workinprogress.oowsection.org/2017/11/14/to-understand-how-families-eat-consider-what-food-means-to-parents/..

Fielding-Singh, Priya (2018). 'Op-Ed: Why Do Poor Americans Eat So Unhealthfully? Because Junk Food Is the Only Indulgence They Can Afford', *Los Angeles Times*, 7 February. https://www.latimes.com/opinion/op-ed/la-oe-singh-food-deserts-nutritional-disparities-20180207-story.html.

Finkelstein, Eric and Laurie Zuckerman (2008). *The Fattening of America: How the Economy Makes Us Fat, If It Matters, and What to Do about It* (Hoboken, NJ: Wiley).

Fishkin, James S. (1983). *Justice, Equal Opportunity, and the Family* (New Haven, CT: Yale University Press).

Fishkin, Joseph (2014). *Bottlenecks: A New Theory of Equal Opportunity* (New York: Oxford University Press).

Flanders, Chad (2012). 'The Mutability of Public Reason', *Ratio Juris*, 25 (2): 180–205.

Flegal, Katherine M., Brian K. Kit, Heather Orpana, and Barry I. Graubardet (2013). 'Association of All-Cause Mortality with Overweight and Obesity Using Standard Body Mass Index Categories: A Systematic Review and Meta-Analysis', *JAMA*, 309 (1): 71–82.

Food and Drug Administration (2014). 'FDA Food Labeling: Nutrition Labeling of Standard Menu Items in Restaurants and Similar Retail Food Establishments', *Federal Register*, 1 December. https://www.federalregister.gov/documents/2014/12/01/2014-27833/food-labeling-nutrition-labeling-of-standard-menu-items-in-restaurants-and-similar-retail-food.

Food and Nutrition Service, US Department of Agriculture (2007). 'Implications of restricting the use of food stamp benefits.' https://fns-prod.azureedge.net/sites/default/files/FSPFoodRestrictions.pdf

Food and Nutrition Service, US Department of Agriculture (2019). 'Supplemental Nutrition Assistance Program Participation and Costs.' https://fns-prod.azureedge.net/sites/default/files/resource-files/SNAPsummary-7.pdf.

Food and Nutrition Service, US Department of Agriculture (2020). 'What Can SNAP Buy?' https://www.fns.usda.gov/snap/eligible-food-items.

FoodPrint (2021). 'What Is Food Justice and Why Is It Necessary?' https://foodprint.org/issues/food-justice/.

Food Research and Action Center (2013). 'A Review of Strategies to Bolster SNAP's Role in Improving Nutrition as Well as Food Security.' https://frac.org/wp-content/uploads/SNAPstrategies_full-report.pdf

Food Research and Action Center (2017a). 'A Review of Strategies to Bolster SNAP's Role in Improving Nutrition as Well as FoodSecurity'. https://frac.org/research/resource-library/review-strategies-bolster-snaps-role-improving-nutrition-well-food-security.

Food Research and Action Center (2017b). 'Supplemental Nutrition Assistance Program (SNAP)'. http://frac.org/programs/supplemental-nutrition-assistance-program-snap.

Fox, Ashley M. and Carol R. Horowitz (2013). 'Best Practices in Policy Approaches to Obesity Prevention', *Journal of Health Care for the Poor and Underserved*, 24 (2 suppl.): 168–92.

Freedhoff, Yoni (2015). 'You'll Gladly Die for Your Children: Why Won't You Cook for Them?', *US News & World Report*, 11 April. https://health.usnews.com/health-news/blogs/eat-run/2013/04/11/the-power-of-we.

Freeman, Samuel (2007). *Rawls* (Abingdon, UK: Routledge).

Fricker, Miranda (2007). *Epistemic Injustice: Power and the Ethics of Knowing* (Oxford: Oxford University Press).

Frieden, Thomas R. (2013). 'Government's Role in Protecting Health and Safety', *New England Journal of Medicine*, 368 (20): 1857–59.

Fuchs, Alan E. (2001). 'Autonomy, Slavery, and Mill's Critique of Paternalism', *Ethical Theory and Moral Practice*, 4 (3): 231–51.

Gastil, John and Peter Levine (eds.) (2005). *The Deliberative Democracy Handbook: Strategies for Effective Civic Engagement in the Twenty First Century* (San Francisco: Jossey-Bass).

Gaus, Gerald (2010). *The Order of Public Reason: A Theory of Freedom and Morality in a Diverse and Bounded World* (Cambridge: Cambridge University Press).

Gaus, Gerald (2012). 'Sectarianism without Perfection? Quong's Political Liberalism', *Philosophy and Public Issues* (new series), 2 (1): 7–15.

Gaus, Gerald and Kevin Vallier (2009). 'The Roles of Religious Conviction in a Publicly Justified Polity: The Implications of Convergence, Asymmetry, and Political Institutions', *Philosophy and Social Criticism*, 35 (1): 51–76.

Gautret, Philippe (2020). 'Hydroxychloroquine and Azithromycin as a Treatment of COVID-19: Results of an Open-Label Non-randomized Clinical Trial', *International Journal of Antimicrobial Agents*, 56 (1): 105949.

Gert, Bernard and Charles M. Culver (1979). 'The Justification of Paternalism', *Ethics*, 89 (2): 199–210.

Gert, Bernard, Charles M. Culver, and K. Danner Clouser (2006). *Bioethics: A Systematic Approach* (Oxford: Oxford University Press).

Goldberg, Daniel S. and Rebecca M. Puhl (2013). 'Obesity Stigma: A Failed and Ethically Dubious Strategy', *Hastings Center Report*, 43 (3): 5–6.

Gostin, Lawrence O. (2014). 'Public Health Emergencies: *What Counts?*', *Hastings Center Report*, 44 (6): 36–37.

Gostin, Lawrence O. and K. G. Gostin (2009). 'A Broader Liberty: J. S. Mill, Paternalism and the Public's Health', *Public Health*, 123 (3): 214–21.

Grier, Sonya A. and Shiriki Kumanyika (2010). 'Targeted Marketing and Public Health', *Annual Review of Public Health*, 31: 349–69.

Grummon, Anna H., Marissa G. Hall, Jason P. Block, Sara N. Bleich, Eric B. Rimm, Lindsey Smith Taillie, and Anne Barnhill (2020). 'Ethical Considerations for Food and Beverage Warnings', *Physiology & Behavior*, 222: 112930.

Guptill, Amy E., Denise A. Copelton, and Betsy Lucal (2013). *Food and Society: Principles and Paradoxes* (Cambridge, UK: Polity).

Guthman, Julie (2007). 'Can't Stomach It: How Michael Pollan et al. Made Me Want to Eat Cheetos', *Gastronomica*, 7 (3): 75–79.

Guthman, Julie (2011). *Weighing In: Obesity, Food Justice, and the Limits of Capitalism* (Berkeley: University of California Press).

Guthman, Julie and Melanie DuPuis (2006). 'Embodying Neoliberalism: Economy, Culture, and the Politics of Fat', *Environment and Planning D: Society and Space*, 24 (3): 427–48.

Gutmann, Amy and Dennis Thompson (1996). *Democracy and Disagreement* (Cambridge, MA: Harvard University Press).

Guttman, Nurit and Charles T. Salmon (2004). 'Guilt, Fear, Stigma and Knowledge Gaps: Ethical Issues in Public Health Communication Interventions', *Bioethics*, 18 (6): 531–52.

Habermas, Jürgen (1996). 'Three Normative Models of Democracy.' In *Democracy and Difference*, ed. Seyla Benhabib (Princeton, NJ: Princeton University Press), 21–30.

Hales, Craig M., Cheryl D. Fryar, and Margaret D. Carroll (2018). 'Trends in Obesity and Severe Obesity Prevalence in US Youth and Adults by Sex and Age, 2007–2008 to 2015–2016', *JAMA*, 319 (16): 1723–25.

Hanna, Jason (2018). *In Our Best Interest: A Defense of Paternalism* (Oxford: Oxford University Press).

Hausman, D. and B. Welch, 2010. 'To Nudge or Not to Nudge', *Journal of Political Philosophy*, 18: 123–36.

Hawkes, Corinna, Trenton G. Smith, Jo Jewell, Jane Wardle, Ross A. Hammond, Sharon Friel, Anne Marie Thow, and Juliana Kain (2015). 'Smart Food Policies for Obesity Prevention', *The Lancet*, 385 (9985): 2410–21.

Hayek, Friedrich A. (1960). *The Constitution of Liberty* (London: Routledge and Kegan Paul).

Hayek, Friedrich A. (1982). *Law, Legislation and Liberty* (London: Routledge).

Hobbes, Thomas ([1651] 1994). *Leviathan, with Selected Variants from the Latin Edition of 1668*, ed. Edwin Curley (Indianapolis, IN: Hackett).

Holtug, Nils (2001). 'The Harm Principle and Genetically Modified Food', *Journal of Agricultural and Environmental Ethics*, 14 (2): 169–78.

Hooker, Brad (2000). *Ideal Code, Real World: A Rule-Consequentialist Theory of Morality* (Oxford: Oxford University Press).

Hornsey, Matthew J., Emily A. Harris, and Kelly S. Fielding (2018). 'The Psychological Roots of Anti-Vaccination Attitudes: A 24-Nation Investigation', *Health Psychology*, 37 (4): 307–15.

Huang, Terry T.-K., John H. Cawley, Marice Ashe, Sergio A. Costa, Leah M. Frerichs, Lindsey Zwicker, Juan A. Rivera, David Levy, Ross A. Hammond, Estelle V. Lambert, and Shiriki K. Kumanyika (2015). 'Mobilisation of Public Support for Policy Actions to Prevent Obesity', *The Lancet*, 385 (9985): 2422–31.

Hughner, Renee Shaw and Susan Schultz Kleine (2004). 'Views of Health in the Lay Sector: A Compilation and Review of How Individuals Think about Health', *Health: An Interdisciplinary Journal for the Social Study of Health, Illness and Medicine*, 8 (4): 395–422.

Institute of Medicine (2012). *Best Care at Lower Cost: The Path to Continuously Learning Health Care in America* (Washington, DC: National Academies Press).

Institute of Medicine and Committee on Accelerating Progress in Obesity Prevention (2012). *Accelerating Progress in Obesity Prevention: Solving the Weight of the Nation* (Washington, DC: National Academies Press).

Institute of Medicine and National Research Council (NRC) (2015). *A Framework for Assessing Effects of the Food System* (Washington, DC: National Academies Press).

Jabs, J., C. M. Devine, C. A. Bisogni, T. J. Farrell, M. Jastran, and E. Wethington (2007). 'Trying to Find the Quickest Way: Employed Mothers' Constructions of Time for Food', *Journal of Nutrition Education and Behavior*, 39 (1): 18–25.

Jacobs, Jr., David R. and Lyn M. Steffen (2003). 'Nutrients, Foods, and Dietary Patterns as Exposures in Research: A Framework for Food Synergy', *American Journal of Clinical Nutrition*, 78 (3): 508S–513S.

Jacobs, Jr., David R. and Lyn C. Tapsell (2007). 'Food, Not Nutrients, Is the Fundamental Unit in Nutrition', *Nutrition Reviews*, 65 (10): 439–50.

Jones, Marian M. and Ronald Bayer (2007). 'Paternalism and Its Discontents: Motorcycle Helmet Laws, Libertarian Values, and Public Health', *American Journal of Public Health*, 97 (2): 208–17.

Jugov, Tamara and Lea Ypi (2019). 'Structural Injustice, Epistemic Opacity, and the Responsibilities of the Oppressed', *Journal of Social Philosophy*, 50 (1): 7–27.

Kass, Nancy E. (2001). 'An Ethics Framework for Public Health', *American Journal of Public Health*, 91 (11): 1776–82.

Kass, Nancy, Kenneth Hecht, Amy Paul, and Kerry Birnbach (2014). 'Ethics and Obesity Prevention: Ethical Considerations in 3 Approaches to Reducing Consumption of Sugar-Sweetened Beverages', *American Journal of Public Health*, 104 (5): 787–95.

Kaufman, Alexander (2018). *Rawls's Egalitarianism* (Cambridge: Cambridge University Press).

Kearns, Cristin E., Laura A. Schmidt, and Stanton A. Glantz (2016). 'Sugar Industry and Coronary Heart Disease Research: A Historical Analysis of Internal Industry Documents', *JAMA Internal Medicine*, 176 (11): 1680–85.

Kessler, David A. (2009). *The End of Overeating: Controlling the Insatiable American Appetite* (New York: Rodale).

Khader, Serene J. (2011). *Adaptive Preferences and Women's Empowerment* (Oxford: Oxford University Press).

Kingsolver, Barbara, with Camille Kingsolver and Steven L. Hopp (2008). *Animal, Vegetable, Miracle: A Year of Food Life*, reprint ed. (New York: Harper Perennial).

Kirkland, Anna (2011). 'The Environmental Account of Obesity: A Case for Feminist Skepticism', *Signs*, 36 (2): 463–85.

Kleinig, John (1984). *Paternalism* (Manchester, UK: Manchester University Press).

Kliff, Sarah (2012). 'Georgia's Shocking Anti-Obesity Ad Campaign', *Washington Post*, 3 January. https://www.washingtonpost.com/blogs/wonkblog/post/georgias-shocking-anti-obesity-ad-campaign/2012/01/03/gIQAZB8HYP_blog.html.

Kogelman, Brian and Stephen G. W. Stich (2016). 'When Public Reason Fails Us: Convergence Discourse as Blood Oath', *American Political Science Review*, 110 (3): 717–30.

Kolata, Gina (2013). 'No Benefit Seen in Sharp Limits on Salt in Diet', *The New York Times*, 14 May. https://www.nytimes.com/2013/05/15/health/panel-finds-no-benefit-in-sharply-restricting-sodium.html.

Koplan, Jeffrey P. and Kelly D. Brownell (2010). 'Response of the Food and Beverage Industry to the Obesity Threat', *JAMA*, 304 (13): 1487–88.

Korn, Ariella R., Erin Hennessy, Alison Tovar, Camille Finn, Ross A. Hammond, and Christina D. Economos (2018). 'Engaging Coalitions in Community-Based Childhood Obesity Prevention Interventions: A Mixed Methods Assessment', *Childhood Obesity*, 14 (8): 537–52.

Kristjánsson, Kristjan (1996). *Social Freedom: The Responsibility View* (Cambridge: Cambridge University Press).

Kuhn, Thomas (1977). 'Objectivity, Value Judgment, and Theory Choice'. In *The Essential Tension* (Chicago: University of Chicago Press), 320–39.

Kukla, Rebecca (2018). 'Shame, Seduction, and Character in Food Messaging'. In *The Oxford Handbook of Food Ethics*, ed. Anne Barnhill, Mark Budolfson, and Tyler Doggett (New York: Oxford University Press), 593–613.

Kumanyika, Shiriki (2005). 'Obesity, Health Disparities, and Prevention Paradigms: Hard Questions and Hard Choices', *Preventing Chronic Disease*, 2 (4): A02.

Kymlicka, Will (1989). *Liberalism, Community, and Culture* (Oxford: Clarendon Press).

Kymlicka, Will (1995). *Multicultural Citizenship: A Liberal Theory of Minority Rights* (Oxford: Oxford University Press).

Lang, Tim and Geof Rayner (2007). 'Overcoming Policy Cacophony on Obesity: An Ecological Public Health Framework for Policymakers', *Obesity Reviews*, 8 (suppl. 1): 165–81.

Langfield, Tess, Rachel Pechey, Philippe T. Gilchrist, Mark Pilling, and Theresa M. Marteau (2020). 'Glass Shape Influences Drinking Behaviours in Three Laboratory Experiments', *Scientific Reports*, 10: 13362.

Larmore, Charles (1987). *Patterns of Moral Complexity* (Cambridge: Cambridge University Press).

Larmore, C. (1996). *The Morals of Modernity* (Cambridge: Cambridge University Press).

La Via Campesina (2007). 'Declaration of Nyéléni', Nyéléni Village, Selingue, Mali, 27 February. https://viacampesina.org/en/declaration-of-nyi/.

Lawton, Julia (2003). 'Lay Experiences of Health and Illness: Past Research and Future Agendas', *Sociology of Health and Illness*, 25 (3): 23–40.

Lee, Lisa M. (2012). 'Public Health Ethics Theory: Review and Path to Convergence', *The Journal of Law, Medicine & Ethics*, 40 (1): 85–98.

Lee-Kwan Seung Hee, Latetia V. Moore, Heidi M. Blanck, Diane M. Harris, and Deb Galuska (2017). 'Disparities in State-Specific Adult Fruit and Vegetable Consumption: United States, 2015', *Morbidity and Mortality Weekly Report*, 66 (45): 1241–47.

Leung, Cindy W., Aviva A. Musicus, Walter C. Willett, and Eric B. Rimm (2017). 'Improving the Nutritional Impact of the Supplemental Nutrition Assistance Program: Perspectives from the Participants.' *American Journal of Preventive Medicine* 52 (2): S193–98.

Li, Meng and Gretchen B. Chapman (2012). 'Why Do People Like Natural? Instrumental and Ideational Bases for the Naturalness Preference', *Journal of Applied Social Psychology*, 42 (12): 2859–78.

Lim, Stephen S., et al. (2013). 'A Comparative Risk Assessment of Burden of Disease and Injury Attributable to 67 Risk Factors and Risk Factor Clusters in 21 Regions, 1990–2010: A Systematic Analysis for the Global Burden of Disease Study 2010', *The Lancet*, 380 (9859): 2224–60.

Linde, J. A., A. J. Rothman, A. S. Baldwin, and R. W. Jeffery (2006). 'The Impact of Self-Efficacy on Behavior Change and Weight Change among Overweight Participants in a Weight Loss Trial', *Health Psychology*, 25 (3): 282–91.

Lister, Andrew (2007). 'Public Reason and Moral Compromise', *Canadian Journal of Philosophy*, 37 (1): 1–34.

Lister, Andrew (2013). *Public Reason and Political Community* (London: Bloomsbury).

Livingstone, M. Barbara E. and L. Kirsty Pourshahidi (2014). 'Portion Size and Obesity', *Advances in Nutrition*, 5 (6): 829–34.

Locke, John ([1690] 1980). *Second Treatise on Civil Government*, ed. C. B. MacPherson (Indianapolis, IN: Hackett).

Loi, Michele (2014). 'Food Labels, Genetic Information, and the Right Not to Know', *Kennedy Institute of Ethics Journal*, 24 (4): 323–44.

Long, Michael W., Cindy W. Leun, Lilian W. Y. Cheung, Susan J. Blumenthal and Walter C. Willett (2014). 'Public Support for Policies to Improve the Nutritional Impact of the Supplemental Nutrition Assistance Program (SNAP)', *Public Health Nutrition*, 17 (1): 219–24.

Luke, Douglas A. and Katherine A. Stamatakis (2012). 'Systems Science Methods in Public Health: Dynamics, Networks, and Agents', *Annual Review of Public Health*, 33: 357–76.

Lynch, J. and E. Bassler (2014). 'SNAP Decisions Health Impact Assessment: Proposed Illinois Legislation to Eliminate Sugar-Sweetened Beverages from the Supplemental Nutrition Assistance Program (SNAP)', Illinois Public Health Institute. https://docplayer.net/3852293-Snap-decisions-health-impact-assessment-full-report.html

Macedo, Stephen (2010). 'Why Public Reason? Citizens' Reasons and the Constitution of the Public Sphere'. Manuscript available at the Social Science Research Network. https://papers.ssrn.com/sol3/papers.cfm?abstract_id=1664085

Martin, Crescent B., Kirsten A. Herrick, Neda Sarafrazi, and Cynthia L. Ogden (2018). 'Attempts to Lose Weight among Adults in the United States, 2013–2016', *NCHS Data Brief*, no. 313: 8. https://www.cdc.gov/nchs/data/databriefs/db313.pdf.

May, Stephen (2003). 'Misconceiving Minority Language Rights: Implications for Liberal Political Theory'. In *Language Rights and Political Theory*, ed. Will Kymlicka and Alan Patten (Oxford: Oxford University Press), 123–52.

Mayes, Christopher and Donald B. Thompson (2014). 'Is Nutritional Advocacy Morally Indigestible? A Critical Analysis of the Scientific and Ethical Implications of "Healthy" Food Choice Discourse in Liberal Societies', *Public Health Ethics*, 7 (2): 158–69.

McKague, Meredith and Marja Verhoef (2003). 'Understandings of Health and Its Determinants among Clients and Providers at an Urban Community Health Center', *Qualitative Health Research*, 13 (5): 703–17.

McKenzie, Richard B. (2012). *Heavy! The Surprising Reasons America Is the Land of the Free—and the Home of the Fat* (Heidelberg: Springer-Verlag).

Mepham, Ben (2000). 'A Framework for the Ethical Analysis of Novel Foods: The Ethical Matrix', *Journal of Agricultural and Environmental Ethics*, 12 (2): 165–76.

Merrill, Roberto (2014). 'Introduction'. In *Political Neutrality: A Re-evaluation*, ed. Roberto Merrill and Daniel Weinstock (Basingstoke, UK: Palgrave Macmillan), 1–21.

Merry, Michael S. (2012). 'Paternalism, Obesity, and Tolerable Levels of Risk', *Democracy & Education*, 20 (1): 1–6.

Meyer-Rochow, Victor Benno (2009). 'Food Taboos: Their Origins and Purposes', *Journal of Ethnobiology and Ethnomedicine*, 5 (18): 1–10.

Meyers, Diana T. (1989). *Self, Society, and Personal Choice* (New York: Columbia University Press).

Mill, John Stuart ([1848] 1965a). *The Principles of Political Economy with Some of Their Applications to Social Philosophy (Books I–II)*. In *The Collected Works of John Stuart Mill, Volume 2*, ed. John M. Robson (Toronto: University of Toronto Press).

Mill, John Stuart ([1848] 1965b). *The Principles of Political Economy with Some of Their Applications to Social Philosophy (Books III–V and Appendices)*. In *The Collected Works of John Stuart Mill, Volume 2*, ed. John M. Robson (Toronto: University of Toronto Press).

Mill, John Stuart ([1859] 2006). *On Liberty and the Subjection of Women* (London: Penguin Books).

Miller, David (1983). 'Constraints on Freedom', *Ethics*, 94 (1): 66–86.

Miller, David (2002). 'Liberalism, Equal Opportunities and Cultural Commitments'. In *Multiculturalism Reconsidered: Culture and Equality and Its Critics*, ed. Paul Kelly (Oxford: Polity Press), 45–61.

Mills, Charles W. (2018). 'I—Racial Justice', *Aristotelian Society Supplementary Volume*, 92 (1): 69–89.

Mintrom, Michael and Joannah Luetjens (2016). 'Design Thinking in Policymaking Processes: Opportunities and Challenges', *Australian Journal of Public Administration*, 75 (3): 391–402.

Modood, Tariq (2013). *Multiculturalism: A Civic Idea*, 2nd ed. (Cambridge, UK: Polity Press).

Mohammed, Shimels Hussien, Hailu Taye, Bagher Larijani, and Ahmad Esmaillzadeh (2019). 'Food Taboo among Pregnant Ethiopian Women: Magnitude, Drivers, and Association with Anemia', *Nutrition Journal*, 18 (19): 1–9.

Monsivais, Pablo, Anju Aggarwal, and Adam Drewnowski (2014). 'Time Spent on Home Food Preparation and Indicators of Healthy Eating', *American Journal of Preventive Medicine*, 47 (6): 796–802.

Morales, Alfonso (2011). 'Growing Food and Justice: Dismantling Racism through Sustainable Food Systems'. In *Cultivating Food Justice: Race, Class, and Sustainability*, ed. Alison Hope Alkon and Julian Agyeman (Cambridge, MA: MIT Press), 149–76.

Moss, Michael (2013). *Salt, Sugar, Fat: How the Food Giants Hooked Us* (New York: Random House).

Mulvaney-Day, Norah and Catherine A. Womack (2009). 'Obesity, Identity and Community: Leveraging Social Networks for Behavior Change in Public Health', *Public Health Ethics*, 2 (3): 250–60.

Mytton, Oliver, Dushy Clarke, and Mike Rayner (2012). 'Taxing Unhealthy Food and Drinks to Improve Health', *British Medical Journal*, 344 (e2931): 1–7.

National Association for the Advancement of Colored People and Hispanic Federation (2012). Amicus Brief, 3 December. https://www.documentcloud.org/documents/560 973-naacp-amicus-brief.html.

Nestle, Marion (2007). *Food Politics: How the Food Industry Influences Nutrition and Health* (Berkeley: University of California Press).

Nestle, Marion and David S. Ludwig (2010). 'Front-of-Package Food Labels', *JAMA*, 303 (8): 771–72.

NHS (no date). School Fruit and Vegetable Scheme. https://www.practitionerhealth.nhs.uk/syndication/live-well/eat-well/school-fruit-and-vegetable-scheme

Niemeyer, Simon (2011). 'The Emancipatory Effect of Deliberation: Empirical Lessons from Mini-Publics', *Politics and Society*, 39 (1): 103–40.

Nitzke, Susan, Jeanne Freeland-Graves, and Barbara C. Olendzki (2007). 'Position of the American Dietetic Association: Total Diet Approach to Communicating Food and Nutrition Information', *Journal of the American Dietetic Association*, 107 (7): 1224–32.

Noe, Alva (2012). 'The Value in Sweet Drinks', *NPR*, 24 September. http://www.npr.org/blogs/13.7/2012/09/24/161277720/the-value-in-sweet-drinks.

Noggle, Robert (2018). 'Manipulation, Salience, and Nudges', *Bioethics*, 32 (3): 164–70.

Nozick, Robert (1974). *Anarchy, State, and Utopia* (Oxford: Blackwell).

Nuffield Council on Bioethics (2015). 'Ideas about Naturalness in Public and Political Debates about Science, Technology and Medicine: Analysis Paper', November. https://www.nuffieldbioethics.org/wp-content/uploads/Naturalness-analysis-paper.pdf.

Nussbaum, Martha (2001). 'Adaptive Preferences and Women's Options', *Economics and Philosophy*, 17 (1): 67–88.

O'Connor, Anahad (2017). 'In the Shopping Cart of a Food Stamp Household: Lots of Soda', *The New York Times*, 13 January. https://www.nytimes.com/2017/01/13/well/eat/food-stamp-snap-soda.html.

Office of the Controller, Philadelphia (2020). 'Data Release: Beverage Tax Revenue and Expenditures'. https://controller.phila.gov/philadelphia-audits/data-release-beverage-tax/.

Office of Disease Prevention and Health Promotion, U.S. Department of Health and Human Services (2020). 'Counting Carrots in Corner Stores: The Minneapolis Staple Foods Ordinance'. https://www.healthypeople.gov/2020/law-and-health-policy/bright-spot/counting-carrots-in-corner-stores-the-minneapolis-staple-foods-ordinance.

Oppenheim, Felix E. (1961). *Dimensions of Freedom: An Analysis* (New York: St. Martin's Press).

Paarlberg, Robert, Dariush Mozaffarian, Renata Micha, and Carolyn Chelius (2018). 'Keeping Soda in SNAP: Understanding the Other Iron Triangle', *Society*, 55 (4): 308–17.

Parekh, Bhikhu (2006). *Rethinking Multiculturalism,* 2nd ed. (Basingstoke, UK: Palgrave Macmillan).

Parfit, Derek (2011). *On What Matters.* Volume 1 (Oxford: Oxford University Press).

Patel, Raj (2009). 'What Would Food Sovereignty Look Like?', *Journal of Peasant Studies*, 36 (3): 663–706.

Paynter, Ben (2019). 'How to Get Teens to Give up Junk Food: Tell Them They're Victims of Corporate Manipulation,' *Fast Company*, 23 April. https://www.fastcompany.com/90338482/how-to-get-teens-to-give-up-junk-food-tell-them-theyre-victims-of-corporate-manipulation.

Paz, Christian (2020). 'All the President's Lies about the Coronavirus', *The Atlantic*, 1 October. https://www.theatlantic.com/politics/archive/2020/08/trumps-lies-about-coronavirus/608647/.

People's Food Policy Project (2011). 'Resetting the Table: A People's Food Policy for Canada'. https://foodsecurecanada.org/sites/foodsecurecanada.org/files/FSC-resetting2012-8half11-lowres-EN.pdf.

Peter, Fabienne (2008). *Democratic Legitimacy* (New York: Routledge).

Peter, Fabienne (2017). 'Political Legitimacy'. In *The Stanford Encyclopedia of Philosophy*, ed. Edward N. Zalta. Summer ed. https://plato.stanford.edu/archives/sum2017/entr ies/ legitimacy/.

Pettit, Philip (1997). *Republicanism: A Theory of Freedom and Government* (Oxford: Clarendon Press).

Pettit, Philip (2012). *On the People's Terms: A Republican Theory and Model of Democracy* (Cambridge: Cambridge University Press).

Pettit, Philip (2014). *Just Freedom: A Moral Compass for a Complex World* (New York: Norton).

Phillips-Caesar, Erica G., Ginger Winston, Janey C. Peterson, Brian Wansink, Carol M. Devine, Balavanketsh Kanna, Walid Michelin, Elaine Wethington, Martin Wells, James Hollenberg, and Mary E. Charlson (2015). 'Small Changes and Lasting Effects (SCALE) Trial: The Formation of a Weight Loss Behavioral Intervention Using EVOLVE', *Contemporary Clinical Trials*, 41: 118–28.

Piscopo, Suzanne (2009). 'The Mediterranean Diet as a Nutrition Education, Health Promotion and Disease Prevention Tool', *Public Health Nutrition*, 12 (9A): 1648–55.

Pollan, Michael (2006). 'Six Rules for Eating Wisely', *Time*, 4 June. http://michaelpollan. com/articles-archive/six-rules-for-eating-wisely/.

Pomeranz, Jennifer L. and Jamie F. Chriqui (2015). 'The Supplemental Nutrition Assistance Program: Analysis of Program Administration and Food Law Definitions', *American Journal of Preventive Medicine*, 49 (3): 428–36.

Poore, J. and T. Nemecek (2018). 'Reducing Food's Environmental Impacts through Producers and Consumers', *Science*, 360 (6392): 987–92.

Popkin, Barry M., Linda S. Adair, and Shu Wen Ng (2012). 'Global Nutrition Transition and the Pandemic of Obesity in Developing Countries', *Nutrition Reviews*, 70 (1): 3–21.

Powers, Madison and Ruth R. Faden (2006). *Social Justice: The Moral Foundations of Public Health and Health Policy* (Oxford: Oxford University Press).

Powers, Madison and Ruth Faden (2019). *Structural Injustice: Power, Advantage, and Human Rights* (Oxford: Oxford University Press).

Powers, Madison, Ruth R. Faden, and Yashar Saghai (2012). 'Liberty, Mill and the Framework of Public Health Ethics', *Public Health Ethics*, 5 (1): 6–15.

Pugh, Jonathan (2014). 'Coercive Paternalism and Back-Door Perfectionism', *Journal of Medical Ethics*, 40 (5): 350–51.

Puhl, Rebecca M. and Chelsea A. Heuer (2010). 'Obesity Stigma: Important Considerations for Public Health', *American Journal of Public Health*, 100 (6): 1019–28.

Quine, W. V. O. (1957). 'The Scope and Language of Science', *British Journal for the Philosophy of Science*, 8 (29): 1–17.

Quong, Jonathan (2004). 'The Scope of Public Reason', *Political Studies*, 52 (2): 233–50.

Quong, Jonathan (2006). 'Cultural Exemptions, Expensive Tastes, and Equal Opportunities', *Journal of Applied Philosophy*, 23 (1): 53–71.

Quong, Jonathan (2011). *Liberalism without Perfection* (Oxford: Oxford University Press).

Quong, Jonathan (2018). 'Public Reason'. In *The Stanford Encyclopedia of Philosophy*, ed. Edward N. Zalta. Spring ed. https://plato.stanford.edu/archives/spr2018/entries/pub lic-reason/.

Rajagopal, Selvi, Anne Barnhill, and Joshua M. Sharfstein (2018). 'The Evidence— and Acceptability—of Taxes on Unhealthy Foods', *Israel Journal of Health Policy Research*, 7: 68.

Rajczi, Alex (2008). 'A Liberal Approach to the Obesity Epidemic', *Public Affairs Quarterly*, 22 (3): 269–87.

Ranganathan, J., D. Vennard, R. Waite, P. Dumas, B. Lipinski, T. Searchinger, and GlobAgri-WRR Model Authors (2016). *Shifting Diets for a Sustainable Future*. Washington, DC: World Resources Institute.

Rawls, John (1999). *A Theory of Justice*, revised ed. (Cambridge, MA: Harvard University Press).

Rawls, John (2011). *Justice as Fairness: A Restatement* (Cambridge, MA: Harvard University Press).

Rawls, John (2005a). *Political Liberalism*, expanded ed. (New York: Columbia University Press).

Rawls, John (2005b). 'The Idea of Public Reason Revisited'. In *Political Liberalism*, expanded ed. (New York: Columbia University Press), 435–90.

Rees, J. C. (1960). 'A Re-reading of Mill on Liberty', *Political Studies*, 8 (2): 113–29.

Resnik, David (2010). 'Trans Fat Bans and Human Freedom', *The American Journal of Bioethics*, 10 (3): 27–32.

Resnik, David B. (2014). 'Paternalistic Food and Beverage Policies: A Response to Conly', *Public Health Ethics*, 7 (2): 170–77.

Richardson, Molly B., Michelle S. Williams, Kevin R. Fontaine, and David B. Allison (2017). 'The Development of Scientific Evidence for Health Policies for Obesity: Why and How', *International Journal of Obesity*, 41 (6): 840–48.

Riley, Jonathan (1991). 'One Very Simple Principle', *Utilitas*, 3 (1): 1–35.

Riley, Jonathan (1998). *Mill on Liberty* (London: Routledge).

Roberto, Christina A., Boyd Swinburn, Corinna Hawkes, Terry T.-K. Huang, Sergio A. Costa, Marice Ashe, Lindsey Zwicker, John H. Cawley, and Kelly D. Brownell (2015). 'Patchy Progress on Obesity Prevention: Emerging Examples, Entrenched Barriers, and New Thinking', *The Lancet*, 385 (9985): 2400–409.

Robinson, Eric, Jackie Blissett, and Suzanne Higgs (2013). 'Social Influences on Eating: Implications for Nutritional Interventions', *Nutrition Research Reviews*, 26 (2): 166–76.

Rosland, Ann-Marie, Michele Heisler, Hwa-Jung Choi, Maria J. Silveira, and John D. Piette (2010). 'Family Influences on Self-Management among Functionally Independent Adults with Diabetes or Heart Failure: Do Family Members Hinder as Much as They Help?', *Chronic Illness*, 6 (1): 22–33.

Ross, Nicole M. V. and Douglas P. MacKay (2017). 'Ending SNAP-Subsidized Purchases of Sugar-Sweetened Beverages: The Need for a Pilot Project', *Public Health Ethics*, 10 (1): 62–77.

Rozin, Paul and Michael Siegal (2003). 'Vegemite as a Marker of National Identity', *Gastronomica: The Journal of Food and Culture*, 3 (4): 63–67.

Rozin, Paul, Mark Spranca, Zeev Krieger, Ruth Neuhaus, Darlene Surillo, Amy Swerdlin, and Katherine Wood (2004). 'Preference for Natural: Instrumental and Ideational/Moral Motivations, and the Contrast between Foods and Medicines', *Appetite*, 43 (2): 147–54.

Sanders, Rachel (2019). 'The Color of Fat: Racializing Obesity, Recuperating Whiteness, and Reproducing Injustice', *Politics, Groups, and Identities*, 7 (2): 287–304.

Saunders, Ben (2013). 'Minimum Pricing for Alcohol: A Millian Perspective', *Contemporary Social Science*, 8 (1): 71–82.

Schmidt, Andreas T. (2017). 'The Power to Nudge', *American Political Science Review*, 111 (2): 404–17.

Schwartz, Marlene B. (2017). 'Moving beyond the Debate over Restricting Sugary Drinks in the Supplemental Nutrition Assistance Program', *American Journal of Preventive Medicine*, 52 (2 suppl. 2): S199–S205.

Schwartz, Marlene B. and Kelly D. Brownell (2007). 'Actions Necessary to Prevent Childhood Obesity: Creating the Climate for Change', *The Journal of Law, Medicine and Ethics*, 35 (1): 78–89.

Schwartzman, Micah (2011). 'The Sincerity of Public Reason', *The Journal of Political Philosophy*, 19 (4): 375–98.

Scrinis, Gyorgy (2008). 'On the Ideology of Nutritionism', *Gastronomica: The Journal of Food and Culture*, 8 (1): 39–48.

Scrinis, G. (2013). *Nutritionism: The Science and Politics of Dietary Advice* (New York: Columbia University Press).

Shahin, Jessica (2011). Letter to Elizabeth Berlin, Executive Deputy Commissioner, New York State Office of Temporary and Disability Assistance, 19 August, USDA. https://www.foodpolitics.com/wp-content/uploads/SNAP-Waiver-Request-Decis ion.pdf.

Shenkin, Jonathan D. and Michael F. Jacobson (2010). 'Using the Food Stamp Program and Other Methods to Promote Healthy Diets for Low-Income Consumers', *American Journal of Public Health*, 100 (9): 1562–64.

Shiffrin, Seana V. (2000). 'Paternalism, Unconscionability Doctrine, and Accommodation', *Philosophy and Public Affairs*, 29 (3): 205–50.

Shwed, Uri and Peter S. Bearman (2010). 'The Temporal Structure of Scientific Consensus Formation', *American Sociological Review*, 75 (6): 817–40.

Siipi, Helena (2013). 'Is Natural Food Healthy?', *Journal of Agricultural and Environmental Ethics*, 26 (4): 797–812.

Silva, Diego S., Maxwell J. Smith, and Cameron D. Norman (2018). 'Systems Thinking and Ethics in Public Health: A Necessary and Mutually Beneficial Partnership', *Monash Bioethics Review*, 36 (1–4): 54–67.

Simmons, A. John (2001). *Justification and Legitimacy: Essays on Rights and Obligations* (Cambridge: Cambridge University Press).

Sisnowski, Jana, Jackie M. Street, and Tracy Merlin (2017). 'Improving Food Environments and Tackling Obesity: A Realist Systematic Review of the Policy Success of Regulatory Interventions Targeting Population Nutrition', *PLoS One*, 12 (8): e0182581.

Skinner, Asheley Cockrell, Sophie N. Ravanbakht, Joseph A. Skelton, Eliana M. Perrin, and Sarah C. Armstrong (2018). 'Prevalence of Obesity and Severe Obesity in US Children, 1999–2016', *Pediatrics*, 141 (3): e20173459.

Skorupski, John (1999). *Ethical Explorations* (Oxford: Oxford University Press).

Skorupski, John (2006). *Why Read Mill Today?* (London: Routledge).

Smith, Adam ([1776] 1904). *An Inquiry into the Nature and Causes of the Wealth of Nations* (London: Methuen).

Springmann, Marco, Michael Clark, Daniel Mason-D'Croz, Keith Wiebe, Benjamin Leon Bodirsky, Luis Lassaletta, Wim de Vries, Sonja J. Vermeulen, Mario Herrero, Kimberly M. Carlson, Malin Jonell, Max Troell, Fabrice Declerck, Line J. Gordon, Rami Zurayk, Peter Scarborough, Mike Rayner, Brent Loken, Jess Fanzo, H. Charles J. Godfray, David Tilman, Johan Rockström, and Walter Willett (2018). 'Options for Keeping the Food System within Environmental Limits', *Nature*, 562 (7728): 519–25.

Stephens, Pippa (2014). 'Food Should Be Regulated Like Tobacco, Say Campaigners', *BBC News*, 19 May. https://www.bbc.com/news/health-27446958.

Steiner, Hillel (1983). 'How Free: Computing Personal Liberty'. In *Of Liberty*, ed. A. Phillips Griffiths (Cambridge: Cambridge University Press), 73–90.

Story, Mary, Karen M. Kaphingst, Ramona Robinson-O'Brien, and Karen Glanz (2008). 'Creating Healthy Food and Eating Environments: Policy and Environmental Approaches', *Annual Review of Public Health*, 29: 253–72.

Stroh, David (2015). *Systems Thinking For Social Change: A Practical Guide to Solving Complex Problems, Avoiding Unintended Consequences, and Achieving Lasting Results* (White River Junction, VT: Chelsea Green Publishing).

Strom, Stephanie (2013). 'Report Faults Food Group's Sponsor Ties', *The New York Times*, 22 January. https://www.nytimes.com/2013/01/23/business/report-questions-nutrit ion-groups-use-of-corporate-sponsors.html?_r=0.

Stuber, Jennifer, Sandro Galea, and Bruce G. Link (2008). 'Smoking and the Emergence of a Stigmatized Social Status', *Social Science & Medicine*, 67 (3): 420–30.

Sunstein, Cass R. (2014). *Why Nudge? The Politics of Libertarian Paternalism* (New Haven, CT: Yale University Press).

Sunstein, Cass R. (2016). 'Fifty Shades of Manipulation', *Journal of Marketing Behavior*, 1 (3–4): 214–44.

Sunstein, Cass R. and Richard H. Thaler (2003). 'Libertarian Paternalism Is Not an Oxymoron', *The University of Chicago Law Review*, 70 (4): 1159–202.

Svendsen, Karianne, Erik Arnesen, and Kjetil Retterstøl (2017). 'Saturated Fat: A Never Ending Story?', *Food & Nutrition Research*, 61 (1): 1377572.

Swift, Adam (2006). *Political Philosophy: A Beginners' Guide for Students and Politicians* (Cambridge, UK: Polity Press).

Swinburn, Boyd A., Vivica I. Kraak, Steven Allender, Vincent J. Atkins, Phillip I. Baker, Jessica R. Bogard, Hannah Brinsden, Alejandro Calvillo, Olivier De Schutter, Raji Devarajan, Majid Ezzati, Sharon Friel, Shifalika Goenka, Ross A Hammond, Gerard Hastings, Corinna Hawkes, Mario Herrero, Peter S Hovmand, Mark Howden, Lindsay M Jaacks, Ariadne B Kapetanaki, Matt Kasman, Harriet V Kuhnlein, Shiriki K Kumanyika, Bagher Larijani, Tim Lobstein, Michael W Long, Victor K R Matsudo, Susanna D H Mills, Gareth Morgan, Alexandra Morshed, Patricia M Nece, An Pan, David W Patterson, Gary Sacks, Meera Shekar, Geoff L Simmons, Warren Smit, Ali Tootee, Stefanie Vandevijvere, Wilma E Waterlander, Luke Wolfenden, and William H Dietz (2019). 'The Global Syndemic of Obesity, Undernutrition, and Climate Change: The Lancet Commission Report', *The Lancet*, 393 (10173): 791–846.

Taylor, Charles ([1992] 1994). 'The Politics of Recognition'. In *Multiculturalism: Examining the Politics of Recognition*, ed. Amy Gutmann (Princeton, NJ: Princeton University Press), 25–73.

Tarkan, Laurie (2011). 'Michelle Obama: Fill Half Your Plate with Fruits/Veggies', *CBS News*, 2 June. https://www.cbsnews.com/news/michelle-obama-fill-half-your-plate-with-fruits-veggies/.

ten Have, Marieke, Agnes van der Heide, Johan P. Mackenbach, and Inez D. de Beaufort (2013). 'An Ethical Framework for the Prevention of Overweight and Obesity: A Tool for Thinking through a Programme's Ethical Aspects', *European Journal of Public Health*, 23 (2): 299–305.

Thaler, Richard H. and Cass Sunstein (2008). *Nudge: Improving Decisions about Health, Wealth, and Happiness* (New Haven, CT: Yale University Press).

The Nutrition Source (2013). 'The New Salt Controversy'. 17 May. https://www.hsph.harv ard.edu/nutritionsource/2013/05/17/the-new-salt-controversy/.

The Nutrition Source (2021). 'Sugary Drinks'. https://www.hsph.harvard.edu/nutritio nsource/sugary-drinks-fact-sheet/.

Thomas, Samantha L., Jim Hyde, Asuntha Karunaratne, Rick Kausman, and Paul A. Komesaroff (2008). '"They All Work . . . When You Stick to Them": A Qualitative Investigation of Dieting, Weight Loss, and Physical Exercise, in Obese Individuals', Nutrition Journal, 7: 34.

Thornton, Pamela L., Edith C. Kieffer, Yamir Salabarría-Peña, Angela Odoms-Young, Sharla K. Willis, Helen Kim, and Maria A. Salinas (2006). 'Weight, Diet, and Physical Activity—Related Beliefs and Practices among Pregnant and Postpartum Latino Women: The Role of Social Support', Maternal and Child Health Journal, 10 (1): 95–104.

Trichopolus, Dimitrios, Pagona Lagiou, and Antonia Trichopolus (2000). 'Evidence-Based Nutrition', Asia Pacific Journal of Clinical Nutrition, 9 (S1): S4–S9.

Trout, J. D. (2005). 'Paternalism and Cognitive Bias', Law and Philosophy, 24 (4): 393–434.

US Department of Agriculture (2007). 'Implications of Restricting the Use of Food Stamp Benefits'. https://www.fns.usda.gov/implication-restricting-use-food-stamp-benefits.

US Department of Agriculture, Economic Research Service (2020). 'Very Low Food Security by Household Characteristics'. https://www.ers.usda.gov/topics/food-nutrit ion-assistance/food-security-in-the-us/key-statistics-graphics/#foodsecure.

US Department of Health and Human Services and US Department of Agriculture (2015). 2015–2020 Dietary Guidelines for Americans. 8th ed. https://health.gov/dietar yguidelines/2015/guidelines/.

US Food and Drug Administration (2020). 'Changes to the Nutrition Facts Label'. https://www.fda.gov/food/food-labeling-nutrition/changes-nutrition-facts-label.

Vallier, Kevin (2011). 'Against Public Reason Liberalism's Accessibility Requirement', Journal of Moral Philosophy, 8 (3): 366–89.

Vallier, Kevin (2014). Liberal Politics and Public Faith: Beyond Separation (New York: Routledge).

Vallier, Kevin (2016). 'In Defence of Intelligible Reasons in Public Justification', The Philosophical Quarterly, 66 (264): 596–616.

Vallier, Kevin (2019). Must Politics Be War? Restoring Our Trust in the Open Society (New York: Oxford University Press).

VanDeVeer, Donald (1986). Paternalistic Intervention: The Moral Bounds of Benevolence (Princeton, NJ: Princeton University Press).

Voigt, Kristin (2012). 'Childhood Obesity and Restrictions of Parental Liberty: A Response to "Paternalism, Obesity, and Tolerable Levels of Risk"', Democracy & Education, 20 (1): 1–4.

Voigt, Kristin, Stuart G. Nicholls, and Garrath Williams (2014). Childhood Obesity: Ethical and Policy Issues (New York: Oxford University Press).

Volkow, N. D., G.-J. Wang, D. Tomasi, and R. D. Baler (2013). 'Obesity and Addiction: Neurobiological Overlaps.' Obesity Reviews 14(1): 2–18.

Waldron, Jeremy (2014). 'It's All for Your Own Good', The New York Review of Books, 9 October. https://www.nybooks.com/articles/2014/10/09/cass-sunstein-its-all-your-own-good/.

Walker, Tom (2016). 'Paternalism and Populations', Public Health Ethics, 9 (1): 46–54.

Wall, Steven (1998). Liberalism, Perfectionism and Restraint (Cambridge: Cambridge University Press).

Wall, Steven (2018). 'Perfectionism and Paternalism'. In The Routledge Handbook of the Philosophy of Paternalism, ed. Kalle Grill and Jason Hanna (Abingdon, UK: Routledge), 170–81.

Wang, Zhiqiang, Meina Liu, Tania Pan, and Shilu Tong (2016). 'Lower Mortality Associated with Overweight in the U.S. National Health Interview Survey', *Medicine*, 95 (2): e2424.

Wansink, Brian (2007). *Mindless Eating: Why We Eat More Than We Think* (New York: Bantam Books).

Weber, Max ([1918] 1991). 'Politics as a Vocation'. In *From Max Weber: Essays in Sociology*, ed. Hand H. Gerth and C. Wright Mills (London: Routledge), 77–128.

Weber, Max (1964). *The Theory of Social and Economic Organization*, ed. Talcott Parsons (New York: Free Press).

Weithman, Paul (2010). *Why Political Liberalism?* (New York: Oxford University Press).

Wickins-Drazilova, Dita and Garrath Williams (2011). 'Ethics and Public Policy'. In *Epidemiology of Obesity in Children and Adolescents*, ed. Luis A. Moreno, Iris Pigeot, and Wolfgang Ahrens (New York: Springer Science+Business Media), 7–20.

Wikler, Daniel I. (1978). 'Persuasion and Coercion for Health: Ethical Issues in Government Efforts to Change Life-Styles', *Milbank Memorial Fund Quarterly*, 56 (3): 303–38.

Wikler, Daniel (1987). 'Who Should Be Blamed for Being Sick?', *Health Education & Behavior*, 14 (1): 11–25.

Wilkerson, Abby (2010). ' "Obesity", the Transnational Plate, and the Thin Contract', *Radical Philosophy Review*, 13 (1): 43–67.

Wilkinson, T. M. (2017). 'Counter-Manipulation and Health Promotion', *Public Health Ethics*, 10 (3): 257–66.

Willett, Walter, Johan Rockström, Brent Loken, Marco Springmann, Tim Lang, Sonja Vermeulen, Tara Garnett, David Tilman, Fabrice DeClerck, Amanda Wood, Malin Jonell, Michael Clark, Line J Gordon, Jessica Fanzo, Corinna Hawkes, Rami Zurayk, Juan A Rivera, Wim De Vries, Lindiwe Majele Sibanda, Ashkan Afshin, Abhishek Chaudhary, Mario Herrero, Rina Agustina, Francesco Branca, Anna Lartey, Shenggen Fan, Beatrice Crona, Elizabeth Fox, Victoria Bignet, Max Troell, Therese Lindahl, Sudhvir Singh, Sarah E Cornell, K Srinath Reddy, Sunita Narain, Sania Nishtar, and Christopher J L Murray (2019). 'Food in the Anthropocene: The EAT–Lancet Commission on Healthy Diets from Sustainable Food Systems', *The Lancet*, 393 (10170): P447–P492.

Williams, Bernard (1981). *Moral Luck* (Cambridge: Cambridge University Press).

Williams, Garrath (2015). 'The IDEFICS Intervention: What Can We Learn for Public Policy?', *Obesity Reviews*, 16 (suppl. 2): 151–61.

Wilson, James (2011). 'Health Inequities'. In *Public Health Ethics: Key Concepts and Issues in Policy and Practice*, ed. Angus Dawson (Cambridge: Cambridge University Press), 211–30.

Wolf, Joan B. (2010). *Is Breast Best? Taking on the Breastfeeding Experts and the New High Stakes of Motherhood* (New York: NYU Press).

Wolterstorff, Nicholas (1997). 'The Role of Religion in Decision and Discussion of Political Issues'. In *Religion in the Public Square*, ed. Robert Audi and Nicholas Wolterstorff (Lanham, MD: Rowman and Littlefield), 67–120.

Womack, C. A. (2014). 'Gender, Obesity, and Stigmatization'. In *Encyclopedia of Food and Agricultural Ethics*, ed. P. B. Thompson and D. M. Kaplan (New York: Springer), 1100–107.

Wong, Julia Carrie (2020). 'Hydroxychloroquine: How an Unproven Drug Became Trump's Coronavirus "Miracle Cure"', *The Guardian*, 7 April. https://www.theguard ian.com/world/2020/apr/06/hydroxychloroquine-trump-coronavirus-drug.

Wood, Allen W. (2014). 'Coercion, Manipulation, Exploitation'. In *Manipulation: Theory and Practice*, ed. Christian Coons and Michael Weber (Oxford: Oxford University Press), 17–50.

World Cancer Research Fund International (no date). 'NOURISHING Framework'. https://www.wcrf.org/int/policy/nourishing/our-policy-framework-promote-heal thy-diets-reduce-obesity.

World Health Organization (2013). *Global Action Plan for the Prevention and Control of Non-communicable Diseases 2013–2020* (Geneva: World Health Organization).

World Health Organization (2017). *Prevalence of Overweight among Adults, BMI ≥ 25, Crude—Estimates by WHO Region: WHO/NCD-RisC and WHO Global Health Observatory Data Repository.* http://apps.who.int/gho/data/view.main.BMI25CR EGv?lang=en.

World Health Organization (2020). 'Social Determinants of Health'. https://www.who.int/ health-topics/social-determinants-of-health#tab=tab_1.

World News Tonight (2020). 'President Trump Touts Unproven Drug as "Game Changer"', *ABC News*, 20 March. https://www.youtube.com/watch?v=xAGLGbcQAPU.

Xu, Hanfei, Cupples, L. Adrienne, Andrew Stokes, and Ching-Ti Liu (2018). 'Association of Obesity with Mortality over 24 Years of Weight History: Findings from the Framingham Heart Study', *JAMA Network Open*, 1 (7): e184587.

Young, Iris Marion (1990). *Justice and the Politics of Difference* (Princeton, NJ: Princeton University Press).

Ziauddeen, H., and P. C. Fletcher (2013). 'Is Food Addiction a Valid and Useful Concept?' *Obesity Reviews*, 14 (1): 19–28.

Zlatevska, Natalina, Chris Dubelaar, and Stephen Holden (2014). 'Sizing Up the Effect of Portion Size on Consumption: A Meta-Analytic Review', *Journal of Marketing*, 78 (3): 140–54.

Index